MW01110121

C.W. Hanke B. Sommer · G. Sattler (Eds.)

Tumescent Local Anesthesia

Springer-Verlag Berlin Heidelberg GmbH

C. W. Hanke B. Sommer G. Sattler (Eds.)

Tumescent Local Anesthesia

With 133 Figures, 121 in colour and 13 Tables

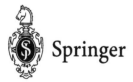 Springer

Dr. C. W. Hanke, MD
Laser & Skin Surgery, Center of Indiana
13450 N Meridian, Suite 355
Carmel, IN 46032, USA

Dr. med. B. Sommer
Rosenparkklinik GmbH
Fachklinik für ästhetisch-operative Dermatologie
Heidelberger Landstr. 20
64297 Darmstadt, Germany

Dr. G. Sattler
Rosenparkklinik GmbH
Fachklinik für ästhetisch-operative Dermatologie
Heidelberger Landstr. 20
64297 Darmstadt, Germany

ISBN 978-3-642-63063-7

Library of Congress Cataloging-in-Publication Data.
Tumeszenz-Lokalanästhesie. English. Tumescent local anesthesia / [edited by] C. W. Hanke,
B. Sommer, G. Sattler. p. ; cm. Includes bibliographical references.
     ISBN 978-3-642-63063-7   ISBN 978-3-642-56744-5 (eBook)
     DOI 10.1007/978-3-642-56744-5
     1. Tumescent local anesthesia. I. Hanke, C. W. (C. William), 1944- II. Sommer B. (Boris)
III. Sattler, G. (Gerhard), 1955- [DNLM: 1. Anesthesia, Local--methods.] RD85.T85 T8613 2000
617.9'66--dc21

© Springer-Verlag Berlin Heidelberg 2001
Originally published by Springer-Verlag Berlin Heidelberg New York in 2001
Softcover reprint of the hardcover 1st edition 2001
The use of general descriptive names, registered names, trademarks, etc. in this publication
does not imply, even in the absence of a specific statement, that such names are exempt from
the relevant protective laws and regulations and therefore free for general use.

Product liability: The publishers cannot guarantee the accuracy of any information about
dosage and application contained in this book. In every individual case the user must check
such information by consulting the relevant literature.

Cover degsin: de'blik, Berlin
Typesetting: Goldener Schnitt, Sinzheim
Printed on acid-free paper   SPIN: 10735754   22/3130   5 4 3 2 1 0

Contents

Part A   Theory

Part B   Practical Application

Part C   Indications

List of Contributors

Dr. med. Matthias Augustin
Dermatologist, Head of the Surgical Department at the
Universitaets Hautklinik Freiburg, Hauptstr. 7, 79104 Freiburg,
Germany

Dr. med. Guillermo Blugerman
Surgeon and Plastic Surgeon, Billinghurst 2192, Buenos Aires 1425,
Argentina

Priv.-Doz. Dr. med. Helmut Breuninger
Dermatologist and Surgeon, Phlebologist, Senior Registrar and
Head of the Surgical Department, Hautklinik of the Universitaet
Tuebingen, Liebermeisterstrasse 25, 72076 Tuebingen,
Germany

Dr. med. Dorothee Bergfeld
Dermatology Department, Klinikum Darmstadt

Dr. med. Robert Ernst
Surgeon. Practice and Day-Surgery Center for Vascular Surgery,
Weizerstrasse 9, 8200 Gleisdorf, Austria

Dr. med. Alina Fratila
Dermatologist and Phlebologist, Head of the Institute for Esthetic,
Dermatology and Laser Medicine, Friedrichstr. 57, 53111 Bonn,
Germany

Prof. Dr. med. Manfred Hagedorn
Chief Physician of the Dermatology Department,
Klinikum Darmstadt, Heidelberger Landstr. 379, 64297 Darmstadt,
Germany

Dr. med. Ernst Hasche
Dermatology Department, Klinikum Darmstadt

Dr. med. Rainer Jokisch
Dermatologist. Dermatology Department, Klinikum Darmstadt

Dr. med. Ralph P. Kuner
Gynecologist and Senior Registrar at the Women's Hospital,
Head of the Department of Senology/Plastic Breast Surgery at the
St. Joseph's Hospital Wiesbaden, Solmstrasse 15, 65189 Wiesbaden,
Germany

Dr. med. Antonio Picoto
Prof. for Dermatology, Centro de Dermatologia Medico-Cirurgica,
Rua Jose Estevado 135, 1100 Lisboa, Portugal

Dr. med. Stephan Rapprich
Dermatologist, Senior Registrar at the Dermatology Department,
Klinikum Darmstadt

Dr. med. Matthias Sandhofer
Dermatologist, Day-Clinic for Dermatological Surgery, Linz, Austria

Dr. med. Sonja Sattler
Dermatology Department, Klinikum Darmstadt

Diego Schavelzon, M.D.
Surgeon, Plastic Surgeon, Plastic Surgery Center, Billinghurst 2192,
Buenos Aires 1425, Argentina

Prof. Dr. med. Wilfried Schmeller
Chief Registrar at the Dermatology Department of the Universitaet
Luebeck, Ratzeburger Allee 160, 23538 Luebeck, Germany

Dr. Stephan K. W. Schwarz
Dept. of Pharmacology & Therapeutics and Dept. of Anesthesia,
The University of British Columbia, 2176 Health Sciences Mall,
Vancouver B. C. V6T 1Z3, Canada

Dr. med. Martin Simon
Dermatologist. Dermatology Department, Klinikum Darmstadt

David M. Spencer, M.D.
Dermatologist, Director, Piedmont Cosmetic Surgery
and Dermatology Center, 3333 Brookview Hills Blvd., Suite 201,
Winston-Salem, N.C. 27103, USA

Prof. Dr. med. Wolfgang Vanscheidt
Chief Registrar at the Universitaets Hautklinik Freiburg,
Hauptstrasse 7, 79104 Freiburg, Germany

Foreword to the English Edition

This book is a product of the German Experience using tumescent local anesthesia for liposuction and other procedures. The German Experience began in 1990, three years after Jeffrey Klein published his landmark article on tumescent liposuction. The centerpoint of the German Experience has been the renowned Darmstadt Live Surgery Symposium directed by Dr. med. Gerhard Sattler. The Symposium has been held in 1992, 1994, 1996, and 1998. The next Symposium, scheduled for November 9–12, 2000, will be directed by Drs. Sattler, Sommer, and their German colleagues. Imagine live surgery performed simultaneously in the operating rooms of a dermatology hospital (Hautklinik Darmstadt) and a separate ambulatory surgery clinic (Rosenpark Klinik Darmstadt) with immediate satellite transmission to the Symposium hotel ten miles away. The four hundred physicians in attendance will have the opportunity to observe and question experienced surgeons during surgery.

This book was published in German in November 1998 as the proceedings of the First Symposium on Tumescent Local Anesthesia (TLA) which was held during the Third Darmstadt Live Surgery Symposium. It contains the experience of multiple surgeons and physicians who have applied tumescent local anesthesia to various areas of medicine. Although I was involved with the planning and execution of the TLA Symposium and the book, the real credit should be given to the German dermatologic surgeons whose brilliance and innovation made this work a reality. These remarkable individuals include Gerhard Sattler, Boris Sommer, Dorothee Bergfeld, and Sonja Sattler. There are many other outstanding physicians who contributed to the book. I would like to congratulate them all for their accomplishments. The readers of this work are invited to attend future Darmstadt Live Surgery Symposia where cutting edge information on TLA and other surgical techniques will be shared.

C. William Hanke, M.D.
President
International Society for Dermatologic Surgery
Indianapolis, Indiana
March 14, 2000

Foreword

It is safe to say that without Jeffrey Klein, who first described tumescent local anesthesia, this book would never have been written. This technique of local anesthesia, originally designed for use in outpatient liposuction procedures in the United States of America, was introduced into clinical practice in Darmstadt in 1990 and is now employed in a growing number of areas of surgical dermatology. Eight years of experience have shown it to be a particularly elegant and safe method of local anesthesia, especially in the treatment of large areas of skin.

A large number of scientific studies have improved our understanding of tumescent local anesthesia. The administration of large quantities of a dilute local anesthetic into lipophilic tissue is no longer seen as a risk to the patient, although further discussion at the international level will be required over the next few years in order to standardize the tumescent solution. Until then, the widely varying dosages reported around the world should be regarded with caution. The progress made and experience gained in recent years make it likely that tumescent local anesthesia will become firmly established in all branches of surgery.

One important factor is the economy of the tumescent technique, the material costs of which are very low. In comparison to general anesthesia, enormous savings can be made in the costs of postoperative care, owing to reduced staff requirements and fewer complications of wound healing.

This book is intended as a guide for those who are either returning to this method of anesthesia or are using it for the first time. We have therefore tried to keep the text as compact as possible, surveying each operative area in turn and listing together the advantages and the disadvantages of the technique for each.

Our thanks go to all those whose work contributed to the making of this book, especially our colleagues at the Hautklinik Darmstadt and the Rosenpark Klinik Darmstadt.

We firmly believe that the increasing use of tumescent local anesthesia will not only attract more supporters of this technique, but will also lead to a multitude of new indications for its use.

We look forward with our readers to the exciting events in store ahead.

The editors, October 1998 and March 2000
Darmstadt and Indianapolis

Part A

Theory

1   Introduction and Definition

B. SOMMER, C.W. HANKE, G. SATTLER

Definition

Tumescent local anesthesia (TLA) is a technique for regional anesthesia of the skin and the subcutaneous fatty tissue by means of direct infiltration of large volumes of a dilute local anesthetic. "Tumescent" derives from the Latin *tumescere*, meaning "to swell," and in this context refers to the swelling of the anesthetized skin after subcutaneous infiltration of the TLA solution.

In addition to the fact that with this method of local anesthesia it is possible to treat large areas of the body which previously could only be operated upon under general anesthesia, more specific advantages have been discovered as experience has grown (see Chap. 8). The great intraoperative safety of TLA and the possibility of immediate postoperative mobilization are particularly worth mentioning.

Target Group

Originated and considerably refined by surgical dermatologists, this method was first taught to colleagues performing liposuction, i.e., general and plastic surgeons and dermatologists, and later to ear-nose-throat specialists, gynecologists, phlebologists, and surgically active generalists. Today many disciplines make use of the multiple advantages of TLA, and each discipline develops the technique further according to its particular focus of interest. The process of discovering suitable new indications continues apace as more and more disciplines gain experience with the technique.

Our intention was to accelerate this lively exchange of information with the present summary of existing knowledge of TLA. For this reason we asked colleagues in various different fields of medicine to share their experiences in this book.

Relevance to Clinical Practice

Our aim is to satisfy the need for information, giving practical tips, not over-glorifying the method, but pointing out disadvantages and pitfalls as well, so as to help simplify the process of identifying indications. All current indications for TLA are listed and presented as a kind of a users' manual, and the individual steps for each procedure are documented with many illustrations.

Outlook

The special features of TLA – its simplicity, its advantages for the patient, and, last but not least, its enormous potential for cost reduction – will lead to a further steady increase in the use of this method of anesthesia.

2 Historical Background

D. BERGFELD, C.W. HANKE

2.1 Evolution of Tumescent Technique

Tumescent local anesthesia (TLA) was developed by the dermatologist and pharmacologist Jeffrey A. Klein, associate professor at the Department of Dermatology of the University of California in Irvine, California. He first described this method of local anesthesia, originally intended to facilitate fat suction in cosmetic surgery, in the January edition of the *Journal of Cosmetic Surgery* in 1987 [17].

The stimulus for this development was the growing pressure on surgical dermatologists in the USA to restrict their activities to outpatient surgery and procedures which could be performed under local anesthesia [2]. It was preceded by the introduction of the so-called wet technique for liposuction (see Chap. 12), a method that had already improved outcomes by introducing large volumes of fluid (saline solution) into the fat that was to be suctioned. The subsequent idea of combining fluid introduction with anesthesia meant that general anesthesia (hitherto unavoidable for liposuction), with all its attendant risks, became unnecessary. Additional advantages for the postoperative patient (see Chap. 8) caused the method to spread and develope rapidly.

2.2 Tumescent Anesthesia in the USA

Liposuction was first performed in the United States in 1980, following pioneering work in Europe by specialists in otolaryngology (Fischer) [6], obstetrics and gynecology (Illouz) [11], and general surgery (Fournier). All operations in Europe and the first ones in the USA were performed under general anesthesia. The early "dry technique" (no fluid infiltrated into the fat before suction) and the wet technique (low-volume infiltration of, saline solution) resulted in extensive loss of blood and marked disturbances of fluid metabolism. Intravenous fluid replacement and autologous blood transfusions were virtually routine with these early techniques.

Liposuction techniques were needed that were safer and resulted in less blood loss. The breakthrough came in 1985 when Jeffrey Klein [13], a California dermatologist, began working with tumescent anesthesia for liposuction. The technique involves small cannulas and the infiltration of the localized adiposities with large volumes of tumescent fluid containing lidocaine 0.05%–0.125% and epinephrine 1:1,000,000–2,000,000 to obtain regional anesthesia and vasoconstriction.

Sodium bicarbonate is added to the mixture to minimize discomfort during infiltration. Most patients can be treated with minimal or no sedation [9]. The blood removed during tumescent liposuction is less than 1% of the aspirate. This compares with 15%–45% using the older wet and dry techniques [8]. Klein's early studies documented safe lidocaine doses of 35 mg/kg [15]. More recent studies have shown that lidocaine doses of 55 mg/kg are safe [18].

Many American dermatologists immediately embraced the tumescent technique because of its enhanced safety and efficacy compared with older methods. In 1991, the American Academy of Dermatology was the first specialty society in the US to publish Guidelines of Care for liposuction [4]. Klein [14] continued with his research in order to refine the tumescent technique. In 1993, The American Society for Dermatologic Surgery (ASDS) published Tumescent Liposuction Survey data that solidly documented the unprecedented safety of tumescent liposuction in a large series of patients [8]. This study of 15,336 patients demonstrated no blood transfusions, fatalities, or admissions to the hospital for treatment of complications.

In 1997, the ASDS published "Guiding Principles of Liposuction" [7]. The standard of care for tumescent liposuction in 1998 recommended limiting removal of fat (exclusive of infranate fluid) to less than 5000 cm^3 in a single session. If additional fat removal is necessary, serial liposuction can be performed.

To date there have been no fatalities when tumescent liposuction is performed in the classic manner described by Klein. Deviation from the classic technique, such as performing liposuction under general anesthesia or heavy sedation, performing multiple procedures during the same treatment session, and using toxic local anesthetic agents such as bupivacaine, has been shown to be dangerous and can lead to serious complications.

Internal ultrasound-assisted liposuction (UAL) requires preinjection of the treatment site in order to prevent burns. The preinjection of anesthetic and vasoconstrictor causes minimal blood loss similar to classic tumescent liposuction. However, there is no evidence to indicate that UAL provides any advantage over classic tumescent liposuction. In fact, the incidence of complications with UAL has been unacceptably high compared to classic tumescent liposuction.

2.3   Tumescent Anesthesia in Europe

Initially, the development of TLA was closely connected to the development of liposuction. The technique of liposuction was revolutionized by the introduction of TLA and the resulting ability to avoid general anesthesia as well as reducing the risk of hemorrhage [16]. The history of liposuction is described in detail in Chap. 12.

A significant European contribution to the development of TLA was the introduction of the wet technique in liposuction by Illouz in Paris [11]. He injected a mixture of saline solution and hyaluronidase into the surgical site to facilitate the suction.

The significance of the TLA solution developed by Jeffrey Klein, which added to the wet technique a local anesthetic, epinephrine, and sodium bicarbonate, was soon realized in Europe. The method spread, especially among surgical dermatologists performing liposuction, partly because dermatologists prefer using local to general anesthesia, and gain much of their experience during training with patients who are awake, i.e. only locally anesthetized.

At first the Klein solution was used at standard concentrations with a lidocaine concentration of 0.1%–0.2%. Because of this relatively high concentration, only 0.5–2 l tumescent solution could be infiltrated during each operation. Since the infiltration was still performed manually with pump syringes, only relatively small areas could be treated in one session. With growing experience, however, it became evident that it was possible to reduce the doses of local anesthetic without loss of effect. The doses of local anesthetic used were therefore gradually reduced from 0.1% to 0.08% and eventually to 0.05%. The simultaneous invention of automatic pump systems for infiltration made it easier to treat larger surgical sites.

The surgical dermatologists found it natural to adapt the advantages of liposuction with the tumescent technique for noncosmetic indications as well [1, 3]. At first lipomas and axillary hyperhidrosis were treated by suction, and the suction cannulas were used for the preparation and mobilization of skin flaps [5].

Lidocaine was replaced by prilocaine at the Hautklinik Darmstadt in 1994. This has many advantages (see Chap. 4). As serum levels of prilocaine are markedly lower than those of lidocaine, this meant that even larger volumes of tumescent solution, up to 3–5 l, could be used [19]. Because prilocaine has a different pH, this mixture also requires less sodium bicarbonate (6 instead of 12.5 ml).

At the same time, other European work groups developed modified mixtures of TLA solution (see Chap. 3). Special mention should be given to the recipes using Ringer's solution (according to Breuninger), which simplify smaller procedures because they do not require additional sodium bicarbonate.

In addition to the changes and improvements in the TLA mixture, the infiltration technique was improved due to growing understanding of the way the solution was distributed in the tissue (see Chap. 9). It became apparent that a lower infiltration rate brought a lot of advantages, but was also very time-consuming. A system was therefore developed which used multiple cannulas at once, each cannula delivering only a small amount of fluid. The advantages of this method are documented in Chap. 10.

The number of studies, clinical experience and the safety and effectiveness of the method for local anesthetization of large areas grew. Improvements in the various mixtures and infiltration techniques occurred and, the spectrum of indications for TLA expanded [10, 12, 20]. At the Hautklinik Darmstadt, TLA was increasingly used in other surgical dermatological procedures, including, beginning in 1993, an increasing number of extended surgical procedures on the venous system. Today, it is used in high ligation and stripping of the long and small saphenous vein, phlebectomy, and, in selected cases, endoscopic perforator vein dissection. TLA has also been successfully used in a large number of procedures that were too extended for normal local anesthesia: extended skin flap techniques, tumor excisions, multiple lipomas, and excisions of extensive diseased areas, e.g., acne inversa.

The tumescent effect of tissue tension has shown to be desirable in procedures such as dermabrasion or split-thickness skin grafts.

The presentation of this method in numerous recent publications, at congresses and continuing education seminars, and, last but not least, the direct experience gained by many interested colleagues learning from pioneers of the method have led to its being adopted in many dermatological departments as well as other fields in the German-speaking countries and throughout Europe as a whole.

The many possible applications of the technique, especially in the field of surgical dermatology, but also in others such as surgery, gynecology, or orthopedics, are discussed individually in Part C.

References

1. Coleman WP III (1998) Non-cosmetic applications of liposuction. J Dermatol Surg Oncol 14:1085–1089
2. Coleman WP III (1990) The history of dermatologic liposuction. Dermatol Clin 8:381
3. Coleman WP III, Letessier S, Hanke CW (1997) Liposuction. In: Coleman WP III, Hanke CW, Alt TH, Asken S (eds) Cosmetic surgery of the skin, principles and techniques. Mosby, St. Louis, 2nd edn, pp 178–205
4. Drake L, Alt T, Coleman WP III et al. Guidelines of care for liposuction. J Am Acad Dermatol 24:489–494
5. Field L, Skouge J, Anhalt T et al. (1988) Blunt liposuction cannula dissection with and without suction assisted lipectomy in reconstructive surgery. J Dermatol Surg Oncol 14:1116–1118
6. Fischer A, Fischer G (1976) First surgical treatment for molding body´s cellulite with three 5 mm incisions. Bull Int Acad Cosmetic Surg 3:35
7. Guiding Principles for Liposuction (1997) Dermatol Surg 23:1127–1129
8. Hanke CW, Bernstein G, Bullock SS (1995) Safety of tumescent liposuction in 15,336 patients-national survey results. Dermatol Surg 21:459–462
9. Hanke CW, Colemann WP, Lillis PJ et al. (1997) Infusion rates and levels of premedication in tumescent liposuction. Dermatol Surg 23:1131–1134
10. Hasche E, Hagedorn M, Sattler G (1997) Die subkutane Schweissdrüsenkürettage in Tumeszenzlokalanästhesie bei Hyperhidrosis axillaris. Hautarzt 48:817–819
11. Illouz Y (1983) Body contouring by lipolysis: a 5 year experience with over 3000 cases. Plast Reconst Surg 72:511–518
12. Jokisch R, Sattler G, Hagedorn M (1998) Vena saphena parva-Resektion in Tumeszenzlokalanästhesie. Phlebologie 27:48–50
13. Klein JA (1987) The tumescent technique for liposuction surgery. Am J Cosm Surg 4:263–267
14. Klein JA (1990)The tumescent technique: anesthesia and modified liposuction technique. Dermatol Clinics 8:425–437
15. Klein JA (1990) Tumescent technique for regional anethesia permits lidocaine doses of 35 mg/kg for liposuction. J Dermatol Surg Oncol 16:248–263
16. Klein JA (1995) Tumescent technique chronicles. Local anesthesia, liposuction, and beyond. Dermatol Surg 21:449–457
17. Klein JA (1988) Anesthesia for liposuction in dermatologic surgery. J Dermatol Surg Oncol 14:1124–1132
18. Ostad A, Kageyama N, Moy RL (1993) Tumescent anesthesia with lidocaine dose of 55 mg/kg is safe in large volume liposuction. Plast Reconstr Surg 92:1085–1098
19. Sattler G, Rapprich S, Hagedorn M (1997) Tumeszenz-Lokalanästhesie. Untersuchungen zur Pharmakokinetik von Prilocain. Z Hautkr 72:522–525
20. Sommer B, Sattler G (1998) Tumeszenzlokalanästhesie. Weiterentwicklung der Lokalanästhesieverfahren für die operative Dermatologie. Hautarzt 49:351–360

3 Composition of the Solution for Tumescent Anesthesia

B. SOMMER, H. BREUNINGER

3.1 Carrier Solution

3.1.1 Physiologic Saline Solution

In the tumescent solution originally described by Jeffrey Klein, the local anesthetic is diluted in 0.9% isotonic saline solution [2].

Note: For intravenous administration the manufacturer recommends a maximum dose of 1000 ml/day; data on subcutaneous administration do not exist. Other medications have been added to the carrier solution in addition to the local anesthetic on the basis of scientifically proven and empirical observations.

The active substances of the TLA solution are added to the saline solution just before administration. The size of the surgical site determines the quantity of TLA solution to be prepared, and the volume of carrier solution is chosen accordingly: for smaller procedures the 1% local anesthetic is added to a 500-ml bottle, for extensive liposuctions to a 3-liter bottle.

3.1.2 Ringer's Solution

Modifications of the TLA solution are useful for the technique of subcutaneous infusion anesthesia (SIA), described in Chap. 10.

The burning sensation felt when physiological saline solution is used can be avoided by using Ringer's solution as the carrier. This means that no buffer solution needs to be added, which simpifies the daily routine of mixing the anesthetic solution and also takes less time. For the same reason no anti-inflammatory agents are needed. Only a vasoconstrictor remains to be added. The concentration of the epinephrine is 1:1,000,000 (0.5 ml Suprarenin 1:1000 in 500 ml solution).

Note: For intravenous administration the manufacturer recommends a maximum daily dose of 2000 ml; no data on subcutaneous administration exist.

3.2 Local Anesthetic

To date only lidocaine (e.g., Lidocaine Braun, Xylocaine) has been used as the local anesthetic in reports of TLA.

We have been using prilocaine (Xylonest) instead of lidocaine since 1994. Prilocaine is regarded as the least toxic local anesthetic, although it does have a tendency to form methemoglobin through its metabolization (see Chaps. 4 and 5). At the same dose, the maximum plasma level is about 30%–50% lower than with lidocaine (see Chap. 4).

3.3 Vasoconstrictors

The addition of vasoconstrictors reduces the blood circulation in the tissue and thus reduces absorption of the local anesthetic. Intra- and postoperative hematomas are much rarer or are smaller.

3.4 Buffer

Adding bicarbonate raises the pH of the TLA solution and thus leads to a higher proportion of undissociated molecules of local anesthetic. This results in better diffusion of the local anesthetic, since only the undissociated part penetrates the tissue. In addition, the H+ ions that cause the burning sensation are buffered, making the TLA solution better tolerated by the tissue. If Ringer's solution is used as the carrier, this additive can be omitted.

3.5 Anti-inflammatory Additives

For several reasons it is beneficial to add steroids to the crystalloid suspension: these not only have anti-inflammatory effects, but also provide a slight psychological euphoric effect during long procedures, as well as stabilizing the circulatory system. Experts differ on the use of steroids in the TLA solution; sometimes, if required, systemic intravenous administration of steroids is favored. Following Klein, at the clinic in Darmstadt we add crystalloid suspension to the solution to extend the duration of effect and to reduce the systemic toxicity [3].

The addition of steroids is not necessary in other dermatosurgical procedures.

3.6 Recipes for Tumescent Solution

3.6.1 Recipes Using Saline Solution

TLA means that dilute solutions of local anesthetic are used to anethetize an area which is swollen by the solution. In reality, there is no such thing as a standard tumescent solution. Even Jeffrey A. Klein, the inventor of TLA, writes in one of his first reports that the concentration of the solution should be adjusted to the clinical situation. He describes three different concentrations: 0.05%, 0.75%, and 0.1%. The higher the amount of connective tissue in the surgical site, the higher the concentration should be. The higher the concentration, the smaller the quantity of infiltrated solution should be. Studies on the pharmacology of the 0.05% solution document adequate intraoperative safety up to at least 35 mg/kg body weight (see

0.05% Solution According to Klein [3] and Hanke [1]. Maximum dose about 6000 ml/ adult

Active substance	Dose
Lidocaine	500 mg
Epinephrine	0.65 mg (about 1:2,000,000)
Sodium bicarbonate	10 mEq
Triamcinolone acetonide	10 mg
Sodium chloride	1000 ml

0.1% Solution According to Klein [3]

Active substance	Dose
Lidocaine	1000 mg
Epinephrine	0.5 mg (about 1:2,000,000)
Sodium bicarbonate	10 mEq
Triamcinolone acetonide	10 mg
Sodium chloride	1000 ml

0.05% Solution According to Sattler [5]

Active substance	Quantity of active substance	Trade name	Dose
Prilocaine	500 mg	Xylonest	50 ml
Epinephrine	1 mg	Suprarenin 1:1000	1 vial=1 ml
NaHCO$_3$	9000 mg	Isotonic sodium chloride solution 0.9% Braun	1000 ml

Note: For use in liposuction 10 mg of triamcinolone acetonide (Volon A 10 crystalloid suspension) can be added.

Chap. 4) (*Note:* The maximum dose recommended by the manufacturer for standard local anesthesia is 5.7 mg/kg body weight for prilocaine and 3 mg/kg body weight for lidocaine). Several common recipes are listed below:

3.6.2 Recipes Using Ringer's Solution

Since SIA can be used not only in extended operations, but also to replace injections in smaller procedures, the concentration of the solution needs to be higher in order to achieve the desired rapid onset of effect, adjusted for the extent of the procedure and the patient's body weight (see Chap. 13). Prilocaine (Xylonest) is regarded as the least toxic local anesthetic, but has a tendency to form methemoglobin when metabolized. Adults tolerate 8–12 mg/kg body weight for TLA and infants and children tolerate 6 mg/kg body weight.

Note: The maximum dose of prilocaine recommended by the manufacturer for standard local anesthesia is 5.7 mg/kg body weight. In thousands of operations in routine clinical practice, three easily mixed concentrations of prilocaine solution have proved effective: 0.1%, 0.2%, and 0.4%.

0.1% solution

Used, e.g., in stripping of veins or in lymphadenectomies with a maximum dose of 600–1000 ml (adults).

> 450 ml Ringer's solution (500 ml bottle –50 ml)
> +50 ml prilocaine (Xylonest) 1% without epinephrine
> +0.5 ml Suprarenin

0.2% solution

Used in children or in extended operations, e.g., scar corrections or sentinel node biopsies with a maximum dose of 300–400 ml (adults).

> 450 ml Ringer's solution
> +50 ml prilocaine (Xylonest) 2% without epinephrine
> +0.5 ml Suprarenin

0.4% solution

Used in smaller procedures with a maximum dose of 150–200 ml (adults), where rapid onset of effect is desired.

> 400 ml Ringer's solution
> +100 ml prilocaine (Xylonest) 2% without epinephrine
> +0.5 ml Suprarenin

The solutions can be used for more than one patient once the end piece of the infusion set (e.g., Heidelberg extension) or the butterfly cannula is changed, since aspiration is technically impossible with the automatic infusion pump. The shelf-life is 2 days if the solution is stored in the refrigerator overnight.

References

1. Breuninger H (1998) Slow infusion tumescent anesthesia. Dermatol Surg 25:151–2
2. Hanke CW, Bullock S, Bernstein G (1996) Current status of tumescent liposuction in the United States. National Survey Results. Dermatol Surg 22:595–598
3. Klein JA (1987) The tumescent technique for liposuction surgery. Am J Cosmetic Surg 4:263–267
4. Klein JA (1995) Tumescent technique chronicles. Local anesthesia, liposuction, and beyond. Dermatol Surg 21:449–457
5. Sattler G, Rapprich S, Hagedorn M (1997) Tumeszenz-Lokalanästhesie-Untersuchungen zur Pharmakokinetik von Prilocain. Z Hautkr 7:522–525
6. Sommer B, Sattler G (1998) Tumeszenzlokalanästhesie. Weiterentwicklung der Lokalanästhesieverfahren für die operative Dermatologie. Hautarzt 49:351–360

4 Pharmacology

S. Schwarz, D. Bergfeld, B. Sommer

This chapter provides a succinct review of the pharmacology of local anesthetics. Emphasis is placed on the two agents currently used in tumescent local anesthesia (TLA), lidocaine and prilocaine. In addition to summarizing their general pharmacological properties, this chapter discusses aspects that are specific to TLA and new issues that have emerged in the course of the advent and clinical application of the tumescent technique.

4.1 Introduction

Local anesthetics (LAs) are drugs that block the generation and propagation of action potentials along nerve fibers. In addition to peripheral nerves, LAs act on all excitable tissues (i.e., central nervous system, myocardium, smooth muscle, and skeletal muscle), an important consideration with regards to their systemic effects (see Chap. 5). Many drugs have local anesthetic properties, including anticonvulsants, α and β adrenergic receptor blockers, volatile general anesthetics, alcohols, barbiturates, opioids, and the biotoxins, saxitoxin and tetrodotoxin. This discussion focuses on the clinically used "local anesthetics", which are aminoesters and aminoamides (see below).

4.2 General pharmacology

4.2.1 Physicochemical properties

Most LAs are weak bases (dissociation constant [pK_a], 7.7–8.9). Typically, the molecule consists of an aromatic head (lipophilic) and an amine tail (hydrophilic in its quatenary [i.e., charged] form), which are connected by an alkyl chain. This chain has either an ester or an amide linkage. Thus, LAs exist as *aminoesters* or *aminoamides*. Examples for the former include cocaine, benzocaine, and procaine. Lidocaine and prilocaine are aminoamides; their structural formulas are given in Figure 4.1.

When brought into aqueous solution, LAs dissociate to form an equilibrium between a protonated (charged and hence hydrophilic) cation and an unprotonated (uncharged and hence lipophilic) free base (Fig. 4.2). Due to this combination of properties, LAs are said to be *amphoteric* (Gr. *amphō*, both).

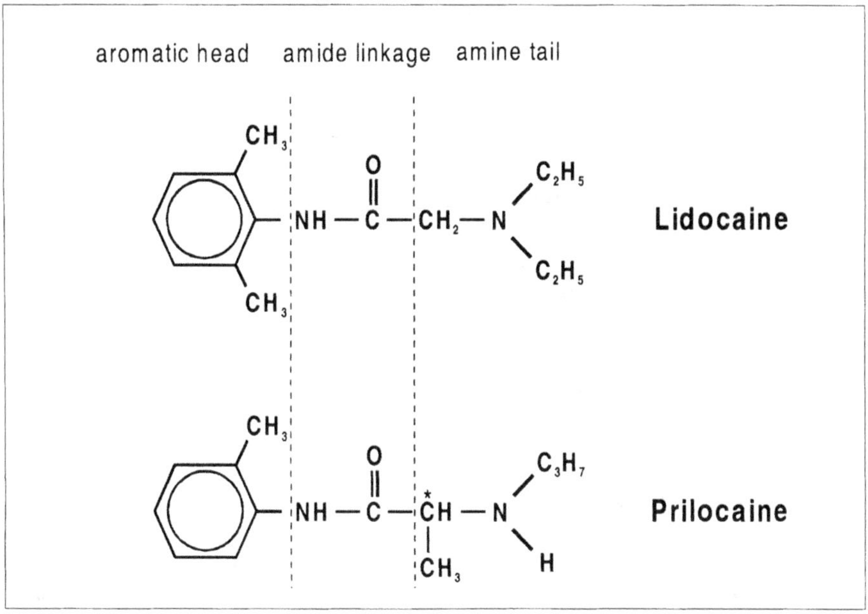

aromatic head   amide linkage   amine tail

Fig. 4.1. Structural formulas of lidocaine and prilocaine. Note that in contrast to the tertiary amine, lidocaine, prilocaine is a secondary amine and also has an asymmetric* C atom. Consequently, commercial preparations of prilocaine contain a racemic mixture of S- and R-isomers, which have distinct pharmacological properties

$$R\text{–}NH^+ \text{ (cation)} \rightleftharpoons R\text{–}N + H^+ \text{ (base)}$$

Fig. 4.2. Dissociation of local anesthetics in aqueous solution

As most LAs are weak bases and the free base is poorly water-soluble, they are usually dispensed as acidic solution, which is more highly ionized and thus water-soluble (e.g., lidocaine and prilocaine hydrochloride salts, pH 4.4–6.4). Once injected, physiologic buffers raise the pH and increase the relative amount of free base present. The lipophilic free base is capable of crossing biological membranes (which is necessary to reach the site of action). However, it is the hydrophilic cationic form that is largely responsible for the pharmacologic (i.e., blocking) effect (see Sect. 4.2.2). The dissociation between the two forms can be expressed as the percentage of total drug in base form and depends on two variables, namely the pK_a of the drug and the pH of the medium. The relationship between pH and pK_a is expressed by the Henderson-Hasselbach equation:

$$pH = pKa + \log \frac{[base]}{[cation]}$$

The pK_a value of a local anesthetic is of considerable significance for its clinical pharmacology. Procaine (pK_a 8.9), for example, is very poorly absorbed from tissues because it largely is present in the cationic form at physiological pH values. Benzocaine (pK_a 3.5), on the other hand, is poorly water-soluble but diffuses well through lipid membranes and therefore is useful only for topical anesthesia. When injected into inflamed (i.e., acidotic) tissue, the effectiveness of LAs decreases, partly because a smaller fraction of free base is available for membrane penetration. Finally, there is a correlation between pK_a and *onset of action*: the lower the pK_a value, the faster the onset of action of a local anesthetic. The *duration of action* increases with the degree of protein binding and the lipid solubility. The lipid solubility also determines the *potency* of a local anesthetic; thus, these agents behave according to the classic Meyer-Overton rule for general anesthetics [35,39]. As well, the more potent a LA, the higher its systemic toxicity (Chap. 5).

The most widely used LA today, both in conventional regional anesthesia and in TLA, is *lidocaine* (Fig. 4.1 and Table 4.1). Synthesized in 1942 by Löfgren and in clinical use since 1947, it is a versatile agent with good tissue absorption, a fast onset of action, an intermediate duration of action, and a good balance between potency and toxicity. *Prilocaine* is similar in many ways; major clinical differences to lidocaine are in its lack of vasodilatory effects and lower systemic toxicity. The latter is compromised, however, by prilocaine's potential for methemoglobin formation (Chap. 5).

Table 4.1. Physicochemical properties of lidocaine and prilocaine [9, 56]

Agent	pK_a	Onset of action	Plasma protein binding (%)	Duration of action	Lipid solubility[a]	Relative potency[b]
Lidocaine	7.8	Fast	65	Intermediate	366	2
Prilocaine	8.0	Fast	55	Intermediate	129	1.8

[a] Octanol:buffer partition coefficient
[b] Data from rabbit vagus and sciatic nerve preparations; procaine = 1

4.2.2 Mechanism of Action

The best-known effect of LAs is the blockade of the generation and conduction of impulses along nerve fibers. At rest, neuronal cell membranes are permeable to K^+, which follows its electrochemical gradient and diffuses extracellularly, leaving a negative charge behind intracellularly. This phenomenon generates the resting membrane potential, which typically ranges between −40 and −90 mV. It is maintained by a Na^+-K^+ ATPase, which actively pumps K^+ back into the cell in exchange for Na^+. Stimulation, i.e., depolarization of the neuronal membrane, produces a short but massive increase in the permeability for Na^+, which is close to zero at rest. If this produces a depolarization of sufficient magnitude at the axon hillock (the "spike generator") of the neuron, an action potential is generated and propagated along the axon.

The principal targets for LAs are the voltage-gated Na^+ channels that mediate the transient increase in Na^+ conductance along the axons of unmyelinated fibers and exposed portions of axons of myelinated fibers (see below). The channels are transmembrane proteins that are selectively permeable for Na^+ ions and exist in three distinct functional states: the *closed* state at rest, an *open* (i.e., conductive) state following depolarization, and an *inactivated* (non-conductive) state, during which the channels are refractory and cannot be activated. LAs act by stabilizing the inactivated state of voltage-gated Na^+ channels [8, 10]. They keep the *inactivation gate* closed, thereby reducing or preventing the depolarization-induced increase in Na^+ conductance [20]. In order to achieve this, the LA molecule interacts with an *intracellular* binding site within the channel. To reach the site of action, therefore, the molecule must first diffuse through a variety of lipid barriers, including the nerve sheath and various membranes surrounding the nerve, and finally the cell membrane (Fig. 4.3). The uncharged form (i.e., the free base; Sect. 4.2.1) diffuses to the site of action whereas the hydrophilic cation produces a major part of the blockade. (Situated in the membrane near the Na^+ channel, the uncharged form also produces a blockade.) These relationships emphasize the

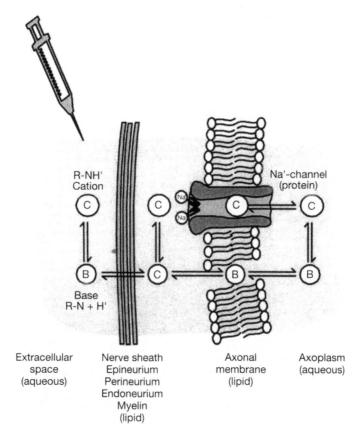

R-NH'
Cation

Na'-channel
(protein)

Base
R-N + H'

| Extracellular space (aqueous) | Nerve sheath Epineurium Perineurium Endoneurium Myelin (lipid) | Axonal membrane (lipid) | Axoplasm (aqueous) |

Fig. 4.3. Local anesthetic access to the site of action

significance of the physicochemical properties of LAs (specifically, their pK_a value; see previous paragraph) for their clinical utility.

Not all nerve fibers are equally sensitive to LA action. Unmyelinated fibers are more susceptible to blockade than myelinated fibers, and small diameter fibers are more susceptible than large diameter ones. The precise reasons for this *differential block* are incompletely understood. The term denotes the clinical fact that pain and temperature sensations (mediated by unmyelinated C and small myelinated Aδ fibers) are blocked before and at lower concentrations than motor signals (mediated by large diameter Aα and Aγ fibers); this property is particularly desirable in TLA.

Besides their efficacy in regional anesthesia, LAs have many other clinical effects, both therapeutic and toxic, some of which will be discussed below and in the next chapter. On a molecular level, it is important to appreciate that LAs are far from being specific agents. In addition to their blockade of Na^+ channels, LAs interact with a wide variety of other membrane-associated proteins, including K^+ channels, Ca^{2+} channels, substance P receptors, and second messengers, to name but a few [8, 30]. The extent to which these actions contribute clinically to anesthesia and analgesia is subject of ongoing research. The contribution of central and supraspinal actions (due to systemic absorption following regional administration) to the analgesic effects of regional anesthesia and TLA also remain in question (see Sect. 4.3.5).

4.2.3 Absorption, Distribution, Metabolism, and Elimination

LAs do not undergo significant metabolism locally in the tissue following injection for infiltration anesthesia or TLA. Thus, systemic absorption and elimination chiefly produce the reduction in LA tissue concentrations. Absorption into the systemic circulation usually requires diffusion through blood vessels walls. Due to the lipophilicity of LAs, this diffusion is rather slow [62], which represents an advantage for TLA. In addition, nonspecific local tissue binding takes place and further limits the fraction of drug undergoing systemic absorption. LA plasma concentrations following local infiltration vary with the site of injection. The highest peak levels are observed after intercostal nerve blockade, followed by caudal, epidural, brachial plexus, femoral, and sciatic nerve blockade. Subcutaneous application yields the lowest plasma concentrations [14]. When assessing LA blood levels, it is important to appreciate that blood and plasma concentrations are not identical and that these may vary with different agents. For lidocaine, the blood/plasma ratio is 0.8, and for prilocaine 1.1 [31].

Following absorption into the systemic circulation, LAs bind to plasma proteins to varying degrees (see below). The protein binding sites saturate at high systemic concentrations, an important consideration for to LA toxicity (Chap. 5) [63, 64]. Besides plasma protein binding, considerable uptake by the lungs takes place and represents another important factor in LA distribution. In addition to the high lung/blood partition coefficient, the relatively acidic pH of the lungs contributes to a buffering function which serves to keep the LAs largely in the cationic form in the tissue (see Sect. 4.2.1) [22,33]. The buffering effect of the lungs correlates with the LA dose and the rate of concentration increase [5].

After passage through the lungs, equilibration takes place between the blood and organs. The concentration in the well-perfused organs (i.e., the heart, liver, spleen, and kidneys) increases initially, followed by redistribution to less well-perfused organs (e.g., muscles and adipose tissue). As a consequence, the blood concentration decreases. Intravenously injected lidocaine accumulates in well-perfused organs after approximately 4 min (reaching higher concentrations than detectable in the blood), and in less well-perfused organs after 16–64 min.

For the most part, LAs are metabolized to water-soluble compounds which are excreted in the urine. The specific pathways for breakdown depend on the chemical class; whereas plasma cholinesterases hydrolyze the aminoesters, hepatic enzymes extensively metabolize the aminoamides, including lidocaine and prilocaine.

Lidocaine

Lidocaine has pronounced vasodilating properties and is readily absorbed by most tissues. Its systemic absorption may be delayed substantially by the addition of a vasoconstrictor (e.g., epinephrine; see Sect. 4.2.5). In vivo, lidocaine is usually 65% plasma protein bound, mainly to α_1-acid glycoprotein. Lidocaine is subject to extensive first pass-metabolism in the liver. It is converted by the CYP3A4 isoenzyme of the P-450 complex and undergoes N-dealkylation followed by hydrolysis. It is important to note that high lidocaine concentrations, as well as other drugs, such as midazolam, diazepam, and sertaline, may saturate CYP3A4. Furthermore, a wide variety of agents inhibit the activity of CYP3A4, including benzodiazepines, SSRIs, cimetidine, verapamil, ethinyl estradiol, and antifungals, to name but a few [28,40]. Lidocaine's chief metabolites are monoethylglycinxylidide (MEGX) and glycinxylidide; both are pharmacologically active. Approximately 75% are excreted in the urine as 4-hydroxy-2,6-dimethylaniline. The clearance of lidocaine, defined as the volume of plasma from which the drug is removed per minute, is 0.95 l/min [62]. Its distribution half-life ($t\frac{1}{2}\alpha$) is approximately 8 min, and the elimination half-life ($t\frac{1}{2}\beta$) is 100–120 min [45].

Prilocaine

Prilocaine does not possess vasodilating properties similar to lidocaine and undergoes somewhat slower absorption. Thus, a vasoconstrictor additive is often not required for infiltration anesthesia. In the plasma, prilocaine is 40%–55% protein bound, chiefly to α_1-acid glycoprotein. The agent undergoes significant pulmonary uptake, to a greater degree than lidocaine [4]. As a secondary amine, prilocaine is not subject to initial N-dealkylation like lidocaine. The agent (particularly the R-isomer; see legend of Fig. 4.1) is hydrolyzed in the liver to yield o-toluidine, which in turn is oxidized to aminophenols. The aminophenol metabolites oxidize hemoglobin and are responsible for prilocaine's potential for methemoglobin formation (see Chap. 5), which has decreased its popularity in conventional regional anesthesia. Compared to lidocaine, prilocaine is metabolized at a higher rate and has a considerably higher clearance (2.37 l/min) [62]. This may in part be attributable to additional metabolism in the lungs and kidneys [16]. Following systemic absorption, prilocaine undergoes rapid redistribution and has a t½α around 100 min. Only 1–6% of prilocaine are excreted in the urine in unaltered form [49]. The slower absorption, high pulmonary uptake, and rapid metabolism result in relatively lower blood levels and systemic toxicity compared to lidocaine and other LAs. These properties likely have contributed to prilocaine's renaissance in TLA, where it is favored by some clinicians. However, at the time of writing, lidocaine remains by far the most frequently used agent in TLA.

4.2.4 Vasoconstrictor Additives

In order to delay systemic absorption, a vasoconstricting agent is often added to LA solutions. This increases the duration of action by prolonging the exposure of the local nerve fibers to the LA (see Chap. 4.3.3), delays the time to reach peak plasma concentration, and decreases systemic toxicity [17, 26, 34, 36, 47]. The maintenance of a balance between systemic absorption and elimination is facilitated and the risk of CYP3A4 saturation reduced (Chap. 4.2.3). Due to its inherent vasodilating properties, the effects of a vasoconstrictor additive are particularly pronounced with the use of lidocaine (Chap. 4.2.3).

The most commonly used vasoconstrictor additive is *epinephrine*. In conventional LA preparations, it is usually added in a dilution of 1:100,000 (i.e., 10 µg/ml) or 1:200,000 (5 µg/ml). The pH value of commercial LA solutions with added epinephrine (e.g., lidocaine HCl with epinephrine 1:200,000) is around 3.5, since epinephrine is unstable at higher pH values and undergoes oxidation [37]. In TLA, the tumescent solution is commonly prepared such that plain LA preparations and plain epinephrine 1:1000 (1 mg/ml) are added as separate components (see Chap. 3) to yield a final epinephrine dilution of 1:1,000,000 (1 µg/ml) or 1:2,000,000 (0.5 µg/ml). Others have used commercial 2% lidocaine with epinephrine 1:200,000 to prepare the tumescent solution [1]. It is important to note that epinephrine itself may produce dose-dependent adverse events as a result of systemic absorption (see Chap. 5). The injection of solutions containing a vasoconstrictor additive into peripheral body parts such as fingers, toes, ears, nose, or penis is contraindicated, as tissue necrosis and gangrene may result.

4.3 Clinical Pharmacology of Lidocaine and Prilocaine in TLA

4.3.1 Concentration of the Tumescent Solution

Before the tumescent technique was introduced, the concentration of choice for lidocaine or prilocaine to produce satisfactory infiltration anesthesia was considered to be in the range of 0.5–2% (5–20 mg/ml) [16, 44]. In TLA, large volumes of

LA solutions diluted by a factor 10 to 20 are used, with a final LA concentration of 0.05–0.1% (0.5–1 mg/ml). Complete anesthesia, comparable to conventional infiltration anesthesia, is achieved with a 10–20 min delay to onset of action. The relationship between onset of action and the concentration of the tumescent solution is such that the time to onset increases with increasing dilution of the tumescent solution. Accordingly, the higher the concentration of the solution, the more rapid the onset of effects. However, this potential to accelerate the onset of effects has a limit and once a plateau is reached, further increases in concentration have no additional clinical advantage [31, 32, 52].

4.3.2 Onset of Action

In addition to the dilution factor of the tumescent solution, a variety of other variables influence the time to onset of action in TLA. These include LA diffusion, lipid solubility, the presence of a vasoconstrictor additive and bicarbonate, and the temperature of the solution.

Following injection, the tumescent solution undergoes local distribution in the subcutaneous tissue by *diffusion*. The rate of diffusion depends on the level of tissue vascularization and perfusion, the degree of nonspecific local tissue binding (only unbound LA can exert its pharmacologic action), the pK_a of the agent, and the existing pH gradients across the biological membranes (see Sect. 4.2.1). The large volumes of solution infiltrated in the tumescent technique and the resulting high tissue pressure facilitate the diffusion of the LA [27]. However, the higher the local blood flow in the tissue, the more LA is absorbed into the systemic circulation and thus withdrawn from the local action. The addition of epinephrine to the tumescent solution counteracts this (see Sects. 3.6 and 4.2.4) [26, 47].

Another important consideration for the onset of anesthesia in TLA is the *site of action*. In the *dermis*, a considerably higher number of free nerve endings are present compared to the *subcutaneous fatty tissue*. For TLA, this has the consequence that surface anesthesia may initially be incomplete while satisfactory anesthesia of the subcutaneous fatty tissue is already achieved. The practical implication is that procedures such as liposuctions may be commenced even when the patient reports some remaining sensation to the skin. A small incision is usually tolerated well in this situation, although some pressure may still be felt. For larger skin excisions, on the other hand, sufficient time should be allowed until complete anesthesia of the epidermis to is achieved. An alternative is to infiltrate the planned excision line with additional 1% lidocaine or prilocaine.

4.3.3 Duration of Action

Prior to the empirical development of TLA, lidocaine and prilocaine were considered to be LAs with an intermediate duration of action (60–120 min; see Sect. 4.2.1) [55]. It was thus thought that their analgesic and anesthetic effects would not exceed several hours. However, the practical experience with TLA has shown that analgesia up to 18 h duration can be produced with the use of large volumes of a dilute solution [25]. The findings of Raymond et al. [43] may provide one explanation for this intriguing phenomenon: they demonstrated that the degree of conduction blockade in single nerve fibers exposed to a constant concentration of LA increases with the length of the exposed nerve segment. In TLA, where large total doses of LAs are exposed to significantly larger areas than in conventional methods of local anesthesia, this mechanism would be facilitated to a maximal degree, resulting in profound and long-lasting blockade of impulse conduction.

4.3.4 Infiltration Rate

As discussed above, the local distribution of LA in the tissue determines the amount of blocked nerve fibers. The LA distributes in the tissue in proportion to the distribution of the infiltrated volume, as determined by the volume of the solution and the infiltration rate [59]. Because large volumes of tumescent solution are necessary, the infiltration rate in the tumescent technique is usually low (see Chap. 10), allowing the LA to undergo optimal distribution in the relevant compartment. In addition, the high tissue pressures that are generated with the use of this technique further facilitate LA diffusion (Sect. 4.3.2). The use of low infiltration rates also has the advantage of decreasing systemic distribution of the LA (Sect. 4.2.3), and hence, reducing systemic LA toxicity (Chap. 5) [12, 13, 16].

4.3.5 Blood and Plasma Levels

In conventional infiltration anesthesia, maximum plasma levels of lidocaine without added vasoconstrictors occur at 2–150 min, depending on the dose and route of administration. Prilocaine peak plasma concentrations are typically reached after 15–30 min [64]. In TLA, where highly dilute solutions are used, the time to reach maximum lidocaine plasma levels is significantly delayed and ranges between 4 and 14 h [7, 26, 38, 65]. This must be kept in mind particularly for ambulatory procedures, as systemic lidocaine concentrations may continue to rise for many hours after the time of discharge of the patient [7]. With few reported exceptions [42], peak concentrations remain below 5 µg/ml, considered by many as the "toxic threshold" of lidocaine (see Chap. 5). For prilocaine, administered at a dose of 35 mg/kg, peak plasma concentrations average 0.91 µg/ml and are reached after 5–6 h [48]. The low concentration of the tumescent solution, the relatively low tissue perfusion, and the slow infiltration rate used in the TLA technique may explain the relatively low plasma levels compared to the large total dose of LA applied. Table 4.2 gives a summary of major differences in the clinical pharmacology of lidocaine and prilocaine for conventional infiltration anesthesia and TLA.

It is interesting to note that the lidocaine plasma concentrations seen in TLA are in a range known to produce central analgesia in vivo [12, 16] and inhibit nociceptive thalamic neurons in vitro [50, 51]. The possibility that the central analgesic properties of LAs [41] contribute to the analgesia observed following

Table 4.2. Clinical pharmacology of lidocaine and prilocaine in tumescent local anesthesia (modified from [59])

Conventional infiltration anesthesia	Tumescent local anesthesia
0.5–2% solution used (5–20 mg/ml)	0.05–0.1% solution used (0.5–1 mg/ml)[a]
Small volumes infiltrated (usually <100 ml)	Large volumes infused (up to several l)

Maximal recommended doses [16]:
  lidocaine with epinephrine:
    7 mg/kg (500 mg)
  prilocaine: 10 mg/kg (600 mg)
	Maximal recommended doses:
	  lidocaine: 55 mg/kg[b] [2]
	
	  prilocaine: 12 mg/kg[c] [6]

Intermediate duration of action (60–120 min)	Long duration of action (18–36 h)

Higher concentration results
  in longer duration of action
	Higher dilution results in longer
	  absorption and longer duration of action

Maximum plasma levels [64]:
  lidocaine: 2–150 min
  prilocaine: 15–30 min
	Maximum plasma levels:
	  lidocaine: 4–14 h [7, 26, 38, 65]
	  prilocaine: 5–6 h [48]

Rate of absorption independent of concentration	Rate of absorption increases with of concentration

[a] Prilocaine also has been used in concentrations of 0.4% and higher [6].
[b] Above recommendation is based on a single study [38] with a sample size of $n = 10$ for the determination of plasma concentrations and $n = 60$ for the determination of signs and symptoms of lidocaine toxicity by telephone interview.
[c] Above recommendation is from a single group of authors [6] and based on their experience with >25,000 patients over 12 years. The use of considerably higher prilocaine doses has been reported by the same group as well as Sattler et al. [48], who reported on the safe use of 35 mg/kg in four patients. At the time of writing, no data exist from prospective studies with adequate sample sizes designed to determine maximum safe prilocaine doses in TLA.

peripheral nerve blockade in the management of chronic pain has been raised previously [3]. No data are available to date on the contribution of central LA actions to the analgesia produced in TLA.

4.3.6 Antibacterial Effects

LAs have antibacterial effects independent of added preservatives [58, 59]. These are enhanced by the addition of sodium bicarbonate [58]. In TLA, where large total doses and volumes are administered, this would represent a potential clinical advantage. The "wash-out effect" that occurs during the first postoperative hours as a result of the tumescent solution leaking from the incisions would in theory further enhance antibacterial effects. However, whereas lidocaine concentrations exceeding 0.8% demonstrably have antibacterial properties, a recent study found no significant effect on bacterial growth of lidocaine, bicarbonate, or epinephrine in the dilute concentrations commonly used in tumescent solutions [15].

4.3.7 Antithrombotic Effects

In earlier liposuction techniques, thromboembolic events were a leading cause of morbidity and mortality [11, 57]. No prospective randomized controlled trial with a sufficiently large sample size has compared TLA to earlier techniques in terms of incidence of adverse events. However, there are only few reported cases of thromboembolic complications associated with the tumescent technique [42]. Local anesthetics have antithrombotic effects in vitro, and regional anesthetic techniques have been shown to be associated with fewer thromboembolic complications than general anesthesia (for review, see [24]). It remains uncertain whether the in vivo effects are indeed due to the antithrombotic LA properties or secondary to other factors such as early mobilization after surgical procedures under regional anesthesia.

4.3.8 Temperature of the Tumescent Solution

Most authors administer the tumescent solution at room temperature. Some cool it down to 4–8° C, and others warm it to about 40° C prior to application [23, 53]. In plexus blockade and epidural anesthesia, the latter results in a noticeable acceleration of the onset of action due to a decrease in pK_a value, and thus a higher fraction of free base available for diffusion (see above) [19, 21]. For practical reasons, it appears reasonable to use the solution at room temperature for smaller procedures. When larger volumes are to be infiltrated, it is recommended to warm the TLA solution to physiologic body temperature. In addition to the potential for accelerating the onset of anesthesia, this may decrease the potential risk of inducing hypothermia, and also reduce the pain that potentially is caused by infiltration of the solution [18].

4.3.9 Shelf-Life of the Tumescent Solution

As discussed in Sect. 4.2.4, commercially available LA preparations with added epinephrine are supplied at relatively acidic pH values, required to keep epinephrine stable in solution. However, tumescent solutions are usually prepared with the addition of sodium bicarbonate, which buffers the solution to maintain a relatively alkaline pH value. As a result, a greater fraction of the LA is present in the free base form, which enhances the effectiveness of the blockade (Sect. 4.2.1). In addition, the chance of an acidic solution producing injection pain is minimized. Nonetheless, this additive reduces the shelf-life of the TLA solution and thus should be added immediately prior to administration. If cooled, tumescent solutions may be used for about 1 day [29, 37].

References

1. Acosta AE (1997) Clinical parameters of tumescent anesthesia in skin cancer reconstructive surgery. Arch Dermatol 133:451–454
2. American Society for Dermatologic Surgery (1997) Guiding principles for liposuction. Dermatol Surg 23:1127–1129
3. Arnér S, Lindblom U, Meyerson BA, Molander C (1990) Prolonged relief of neuralgia after regional anesthetic blocks. A call for further experimental and systemic clinical studies. Pain 43:287–297
4. Arthur GR (1981) Distribution and elimination of local anaesthetic agents: The role of lung, liver, and kidney. PhD dissertation, The University of Edinburgh
5. Arthur GR (1987) Pharmacokinetics of local anesthetics. In: Strichartz GR (ed) Handbook of Experimental Pharmacology, Vol. 81: Local Anesthetics. Springer-Verlag, Berlin, pp 165–186
6. Breuninger H, Wehner-Caroli (1998) Slow infusion tumescent anesthesia – a review of 86 patients. Dermatol Surg 24:759–763
7. Burk RW III, Guzman-Stein G, Vasconez LO (1996) Lidocaine and epinephrine levels in tumescent technique liposuction. Plast Reconstr Surg 97:1379–1384
8. Butterworth JF IV, Strichartz GR (1990) Molecular mechanisms of local anesthesia: a review. Anesthesiology 72:711–734
9. Carpenter RL, Mackey DC (1992) Local anesthetics. In: Barash PG, Cullen BF, Stoelting RK (eds) Clinical Anesthesia, 2nd Edition. Lippincott, Philadelphia, pp 509–541
10. Catterall WA (1987) Common modes of drug action on Na^+ channels: local anesthetics, antiarrhythmics and anticonvulsants. Trends Pharmacol Sci 8:57–65
11. Christman KD (1986) Death following suction lipectomy and abdominoplasty. Plast Reconstr Surg 78:428
12. Covino BG (1987) Toxicity and systemic effects of local anesthetic agents. In: Strichartz GA (ed) Handbook of Experimental Pharmacology, Vol. 81: Local Anesthetics. Springer-Verlag, Berlin, pp 187–212
13. Covino BG (1988) Clinical pharmacology of local anesthetic agents. In: Cousins MJ, Bridenbaugh PO (eds) Neural Blockade in Clinical Anesthesia and Management of Pain, 2nd Edition. Lippincott, Philadelphia, pp 111–144
14. Covino BG, Vassallo HG (1976) Local Anesthetics, Mechanism of Action and Clinical Use. Grune and Stratton, New York
15. Craig SB, Concannon MJ, McDonald GA, Puckett CL (1999) The antibacterial effects of tumescent liposuction fluid. Plast Reconstr Surg 103:666–670
16. de Jong RH (1994) Local Anesthetics. Mosby, St. Louis
17. Eisenach JC, Grice SC, Dewan DM (1987) Epinephrine enhances analgesia produced by epidural bupivacaine during labor. Anesth Analg 66:447–451
18. Fialkor JA, MCDougall EP (1996) Warmed local anesthetic reduces pain on infiltration. Ann Plast Surg 36:11–13
19. Heath PJ, Brownlie GS, Herrick MJ (1990) Latency of brachial plexus block – the effect on onset time of warming local anaesthetic solutions. Anaesthesia 45:297–301
20. Hille B (1966) Common mode of action of three agents that decrease the transient change in sodium permeability in nerves. Nature 210:1220–1222
21. Janik R, Erdmann K, Dick W (1987) Bupivacain-CO_2 und Bupivacain-HCl mit unterschiedlicher Injektionstemperatur zur Periduralanästhesie bei extrakorporaler Stoßwellenlithotrypsie. Reg Anaesth 10:82–87
22. Jorfeldt L, Lewis DH, Löfström B, Post C (1979) Lung uptake of lidocaine in healthy volunteers. Acta Anaesthesiol Scand 23:567–571
23. Kaplan B, Moy RL (1996) Comparison of room temperature and warmed local anesthesia solution for tumescent liposuction. A randomized double-blind study. Dermatol Surg 22:707–709
24. Kehlet H (1988) Modification of responses to surgery by neural blockade: clinical implications. In: Cousins MJ, Bridenbaugh PO (eds) Neural Blockade in Clinical Anesthesia and Management of Pain, 2nd Edition. Lippincott, Philadelphia, pp 145–188

25. Klein JA (1990) Tumescent technique for regional anesthesia permits lidocaine doses of 35 mg/kg for liposuction surgery. J Dermatol Surg Oncol 16:248–263
26. Klein JA (1992) Tumescent technique for local anesthesia improves safety in large volume liposuction. Plast Reconstr Surg 92:1085–1098
27. Klein JA (1997) Anesthesia for dermatologic cosmetic surgery. In: Coleman WP, Hanke CW, Alt TH, Asken S (eds) Cosmetic Surgery of the Skin, 2nd Edition. Mosby, St. Louis, Baltimore, pp 62–70
28. Klein JA, Kassarjdian N (1997) Lidocaine toxicity with tumescent liposuction. A case report of probable drug interactions. Dermatol Surg 23:1169–1174
29. Larson PO, Ragi G, Swandby M, Darcey B, Polzin G, Carey P (1991) Stability of buffered lidocaine and epinephrine used for local anesthesia. J Dermatol Surg Oncol 17:411–414
30. Li YM, Wingrove DE, Phon Too H, Marnerakis M, Stimson ER, Strichartz GR, Maggio JE (1995) Local anesthetics inhibit substance P binding and evoked increases in intracellular Ca^{2+}. Anesthesiology 82:166–173
31. Lipfert P (1995) Pharmakologie von Lokalanästhetika. In: Doenicke A, Kettler D, List WF, Radke J, Tarnow J (eds) Anästhesiologie, 7th Edition. Springer, Berlin Heidelberg, pp 232–272
32. Littlewood DG, Buckeley P, Covino BG, Scott DB, Wilson J (1979) Comparative study of various local anaesthetic solutions in extradural block in labour. Br J Anaesth 51:47S–51S
33. Löfström JB (1978) Tissue distribution of local anesthetics with special reference to the lung. Int Anesthesiol Cli 16:53–71
34. Martin R, Lamarche Y, Tetreault L (1981) Comparison of the clinical effectiveness of lidocaine hydrocarbonate and lidocaine hydrochloride with and without epinephrine in epidural anaesthesia. Can Anaesth Soc J 28:217–223
35. Meyer HH (1899) Welche Eigenschaft der Anästhetica bedingt ihre narkotische Wirkung? Naunyn Schmiedebergs Arch Exp Path Pharmacol 42:108–119
36. Moir DD, Slater PJ, Thorburn J, McLaren R, Moodie J (1976) Extradural analgesia in obstetrics: a controlled trial of carbonated lignocaine and bupivacaine hydrochloride with or without adrenaline. Br J Anaesth 48:129–135
37. Murakami CS, Odland PB, Ross BK (1994) Buffered local anesthetics and epinephrine degradation. J Dermatol Surg Oncol 20:192–195
38. Ostad A, Kageyama N, Moy RL (1996) Tumescent anesthesia with a lidocaine dose of 55 mg/kg is safe for liposuction. Dermatol Surg 22:921–927
39. Overton E (1901) Studien über die Narkose. Gustav Fischer Verlag, Jena
40. Parkinson A (1996) Biotransformation of xenobiotics. In: Klaassen CD (ed) Casarett & Doull's Toxicology: The Basic Science of Poisons, 5th Edition. McGraw-Hill, New York, pp 113–186
41. Peterson CG (1955) Neuropharmacology of procaine. II. Central nervous actions. Anesthesiology 16: 976–993
42. Rao RB, Ely SF, Hoffmann RS (1999) Deaths related to liposuction. New Engl J Med 340:1471–1475
43. Raymond SA, Steffensen SC, Gugino LD, Strichartz GR (1989) The role of length of nerve exposed to local anesthetics in impulse blocking action. Anesth Analg 68:563–570
44. Ritchie JM, Greene NM (1985) General pharmacology of local anesthetics. In: Gilman AG, Goodman LS (eds) The Pharmacological Basis of Therapeutics, 7th Edition. Macmillan Publishing, New York, pp 302–321
45. Roden DM (1996) Antiarrhythmic drugs. In: Hardman JG, Limbird LE, Molinoff PB, Ruddon RW, Goodman Gilman A (eds) Goodman and Gilman's The Pharmacological Basis of Therapeutics, 9th Edition. McGraw-Hill, New York, pp 839–874
46. Routledge PA, Barchowsky A, Bjornsson TD, Kitchell BB, Shand DG (1980) Lidocaine plasma protein binding. Clin Pharmacol Ther 27:347–351
47. Rubin JP, Bierman C, Rosow CE, Arthur GR, Chang Y, Courtiss EH, May JW Jr (1999) The tumescent technique: the effect of high tissue pressure and dilute epinephrine on absorption of lidocaine. Plast Reconstr Surg 103:997–1002
48. Sattler G, Rapprich S, Hagedorn M (1997) Tumeszenz-Lokalanästhesie. Untersuchungen zur Pharmakokinetik von Prilocain. Z Hautkr 72:522–525
49. Savarese JJ, Covino BG (1986) Basic and clinical pharmacology of local anesthetic drugs. In: Miller RD (ed) Anesthesia, 2nd Edition. Churchill Livingstone, New York, pp 986–1013

50. Schwarz SKW, Puil E (1998) Analgesic and sedative concentrations of lignocaine shunt tonic and burst firing in thalamocortical neurones. Br J Pharmacol 124:1633–1642
51. Schwarz SKW, Puil E (1999) Lidocaine produces a shunt in rat thalamocortical neurons, unaffected by GABA$_A$ receptor blockade. Neurosci Lett 269:25–28
52. Scott DB, McClure JH, Giasi RM, Seo J, Covino BG (1980) Effects of concentration of local anaesthetic drugs in extradural block. Br J Anaesth 52:1033–1037
53. Shiffman M (1997) Evaluation of solution temperature for local tumescent anesthesia (letter to the editor). Dermatol Surg 23:309
54. Sommer B, Sattler G (1998) Tumeszenzlokalanästhesie. Weiterentwicklung der Lokalanästhesieverfahren für die operative Dermatologie. Hautarzt 49:351–360
55. Strichartz GR, Berde CB (1994) Local anesthetics. In: Miller RD (ed) Anesthesia, 4th Edition. Churchill Livingstone, New York, pp 489–521
56. Strichartz GR, Sanchez V, Arthur GR, Chafetz R, Martin D (1990) Fundamental properties of local anesthetics. II. Measured octanol:buffer partition coefficients and pK$_a$ values of clinically used drugs. Anesth Analg 71:158–170
57. Teimourian B, Rogers WB (1989) A national survey of complications associated with suction lipectomy: a comparative study. Plast Reconstr Surg 84:628–631
58. Thompson KD, Welykyj S, Massa MC (1993) Antibacterial activity of lidocaine in combination with a bicarbonate buffer. J Dermatol Surg Oncol 19:216–220
59. Tryba M (1989) Pharmakologie und Toxikologie der Lokalanästhetika – klinische Bedeutung. Reprint from: Tryba M, Zenz M (ed) Regionalanästhesie, 3rd Edition. Gustav Fischer Verlag, Stuttgart
60. Tryba M (1993) Lokalanästhetika. In: Zenz M, Jurna I (eds) Lehrbuch der Schmerztherapie. Wissenschaftliche Verlagsgesellschaft mbH Stuttgart, pp 167–178
61. Tucker GT (1986) Pharmacokinetics of local anesthetics. Br J Anaesth 58:717–731
62. Tucker GT (1989) Local anaesthetic drugs – mode of action and pharmacokinetics. In: Nimmo WS, Smith G (eds) Anaesthesia. Blackwell, Oxford, pp 983–1010
63. Tucker GT, Mather LE (1975) Pharmacology of local anaesthetic agents. Pharmacokinetics of local anaesthetic agents. Br J Anaesth 47:213–224
64. Tucker GT, Mather LE (1988) Properties, absorption, and disposition of local anesthetic agents. In: Cousins MJ, Bridenbaugh PO (eds) Neural Blockade in Clinical Anesthesia and Management of Pain, 2nd Edition. Lippincott, Philadelphia, pp 47–110
65. Zhao Y, Song Y, Xue F (1997) A pharmacokinetic study of lidocaine in patients undergoing liposuction with tumescent technique. (Chinese) Chung Hua Cheng Hsing Shao Shang Wai Ko Tsa Chih (Chinese Journal of Plastic Surgery and Burns) 13:63–65

5   Toxicology

S. Schwarz, S. Rapprich

This chapter gives a short overview on local anesthetic (LA) toxicity with emphasis on lidocaine and prilocaine and special consideration of the tumescent technique. The reader is also referred to the previous chapter, which discusses important pharmacologic factors pertinent to LA toxicity.

Toxic reactions to LAs can be classified into the following categories:
- Systemic toxicity
- Local tissue toxicity
- Hypersensitivity reactions
- Methemoglobin formation

5.1   Systemic Toxicity

The incidence of systemic toxic reactions correlates closely with the plasma concentration of the LA (Fig. 5.1). However, the total dose administered may be less

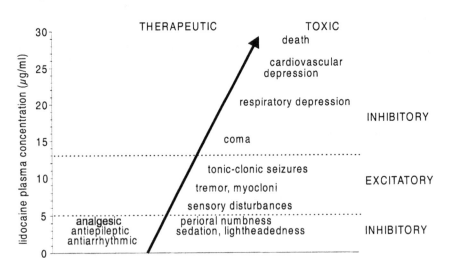

Fig. 5.1 Systemic effects of lidocaine (modified from [3, 6, 17]). A plasma concentration of 5 µg/ml is considered by many the "toxic threshold" for lidocaine. However, systemic toxicity, including the most common symptoms, sedation and drowsiness, may occur at lower concentrations. The same low concentrations also produce lidocaine's systemic therapeutic effects.

significant than the rate of rise of the plasma concentration. The tumescent technique exposes this aspect, because the slow administration of the large total doses in TLA usually produces little signs or symptoms of toxicity, compared to used rapid intravenous bolus injection of considerably smaller doses. Other factors that determine the incidence of toxic reactions include the specific agent used, the pH and p_aCO_2 of the tissue, serum K^+ concentration, and individual factors related to the patient.

In the plasma, lidocaine and prilocaine are largely protein-bound (Sect. 4.2.3). Systemic side effects correlate more closely with the amount of free, unbound drug than with the total LA concentration in the blood. At high systemic concentrations, the protein binding sites saturate and the free (unbound) fraction increases accordingly [18,19]. It is the free fraction that mainly is responsible for the systemic toxic effects of LAs. Systemic LA toxicity emphasizes on two organ systems, the *CNS* and the *cardiovascular system*. The latter is much more resistant to LAs than the CNS, which is the focus of the majority of signs and symptoms of systemic LA toxicity encountered in the clinical setting.

5.1.1 CNS Reactions

Lidocaine and prilocaine both pass the blood-brain-barrier, and high concentrations are reached rapidly in the CNS. The CNS effects are concentration-dependent (Fig. 5.1). Lower, "subconvulsive" concentrations (typically between 1 and 5 μg/ml lidocaine) produce inhibitory effects in the CNS. Patients experience sedation, drowsiness, and lightheadedness, which are the most frequently observed, yet often overlooked initial symptoms of lidocaine's CNS toxicity [5]. At the same low concentrations, lidocaine also has therapeutic properties, including systemic analgesia, and, somewhat paradoxically, anticonvulsive activity (for review, see [7]). Higher plasma concentrations produce excitatory effects. Initial alterations in sensorium (e.g., tinnitus, blurred vision, a "funny" metallic taste) are followed by motor phenomena, including tremor, shivering, myocloni, and, ultimately, the classic generalized tonic-clonic seizures. Further elevations in plasma concentration produce generalized depression, unconsciousness, cardiorespiratory arrest, and ultimately, death.

Whereas the best therapeutic approach to CNS toxicity is prevention, treatment is primarily targeted to maintain oxygenation by means of airway management and administration of oxygen. Seizures are often short-lived; prolonged epileptic activity may be treated with succinylcholine, benzodiazepines (e.g., diazepam), and/or barbiturates (e.g., sodium thiopental) [3].

5.1.2 Cardiovascular Reactions

LAs exert a direct negative inotropic effect on the myocardium in a concentration-dependent manner. This may result in a significant decrease in myocardial contractility, and, in extreme cases, massive hypotension and cardiovascular collapse. Most frequently, however, LAs produce abnormalities in the electrical conduction in the heart. Whereas low concentrations have therapeutic antiarrhythmic (but also proarrhythmic) properties (Fig. 5.1), higher concentrations result in a slowing of impulse conduction. As a consequence, various EKG changes may manifest, ranging from QRS widening to total AV blockade. Clinically, bradycardia and hypotension may be noted. Finally, LAs have direct effects on the peripheral vasculature and at high concentrations produce profound peripheral vasodilation, leading to hypotension, and eventually, cardiovascular collapse [3, 5, 6, 7, 15, 17].

There are considerable differences among the various LAs concerning their cardiovascular toxicity. Prilocaine has favorable qualities in this respect. In terms of its cardiovascular effects, the agent has a low relative toxic potency compared to lidocaine (RTP= dose/lidocaine plasma level/analgesic potency × dose/plasma level of the compared substance).

Treatment of cardiovascular toxicity is directed by the individual clinical situation. In addition to airway control and administration of oxygen, catecholamines, atropine, antiarrhythmics (e.g., bretylium for ventricular arrhythmias), and/or electrical therapy (cardioversion, defibrillation, or pacing) may be necessary [3, 17]

5.2   Local Tissue Toxicity

LAs have the potential to produce direct neurotoxicity and irreversible conduction blockade following injection in the local tissue [3, 17]. This rare complication is usually a result of the administration of exceedingly high concentrations and seems less likely to occur in TLA, where highly dilute solutions are infiltrated. However, although not systematically studied, it is possible that permanent nerve damage due to neural ischemia may result from local pressure from the infused tumescent solution, and careful postoperative monitoring of the patient is advisable.

5.3   Hypersensitivity Reactions

Hypersensitivity reactions (including anaphylaxis) to local anesthetics usually fall into one of the following three categories:
• Reactions to para-aminobenzoic acid (PABA), an aminoester metabolite
• Reactions to methylparaben, a preservative (structurally similar to PABA)
• Reactions to sulfites (e.g., sodium metabisulfite), a group of antioxidants

Compared to the aminoesters, hypersensitivity reactions to aminoamides (including lidocaine and prilocaine) are quite rare and limited to a few single case reports. One should note, however, that multi-use vials frequently contain the preservative, methylparaben, which can cause allergic reactions. In general, the severity of the allergic reactions does not correlate with to the applied dose. Caution is also required in patients with allergies to sulfites. It is important to identify these individuals by taking a careful history and administer sulfite-free drug preparations accordingly.

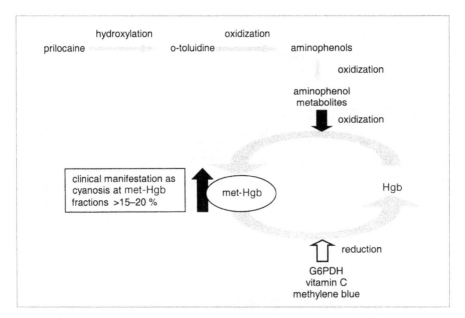

Fig. 5.2   Methemoglobin formation due to prilocaine

5.4   Methemoglobin Formation

Mild degrees of methemoglobin formation have been reported following administration of lidocaine [8]. Prilocaine, however, has the potential for clinically significant methemoglobinemia and consistently causes marked cyanosis in predisposed patients (see below). Prilocaine undergoes hepatic hydroxylation to o-toluidine (see Sect. 4.2.3). o-Toluidine is oxidized to form aminophenols, which are subject to further oxidation. The aminophenol metabolites oxidize hemoglobin and ultimately are responsible for prilocaine's potential for methemoglobin formation, which usually occurs at prilocaine doses exceeding 8 mg/kg (Fig. 5.2.) [4, 7, 12, 15].

Glucose-6-phosphate-dehydrogenase (G6PDH) in the red blood cells physiologically reduces methemoglobin back to hemoglobin. Therefore, special caution with prilocaine is warranted in patients with G6PDH deficiency, an X-linked recessive disorder that affects 5–20% of Southern European and African American males. Similarly, patients with sickle-cell anemia and other hemoglobinopathies carry the potential for an increased susceptibility to prilocaine-induced methemoglobinemia. Due to the immaturity of the enzymatic reduction of methemoglobin to hemoglobin in newborns, prilocaine has practically vanished from obstetric and neonatal anesthesia.

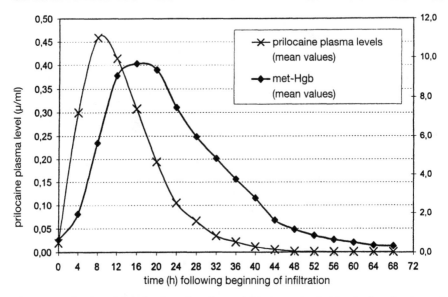

Fig. 5.3. Prilocaine plasma levels and methemoglobin formation in TLA [16]. At fractions of 15–20%, the methemoglobinemia usually produces clinically significant cyanosis. However, this rarely is of further clinical relevance. The cyanosis can be treated with intravenous methylene blue (1–2 mg/kg) or vitamin C (2 mg/kg), which enhances the reduction of methemoglobin to hemoglobin.

At prilocaine doses over 600 mg, methemoglobin fractions may increase to 25%. The fact that a methemoglobin fraction of 10% reduces a hemoglobin concentration of 120 g/l merely to values around 108 g/l may explain why only very few serious complications arise. Patients with a healthy cardiovascular system will usually tolerate this without significant problems.

In one study on the use of prilocaine in TLA, doses of 23–40 mg/kg produced maximal methemoglobin levels of 4.4%–21.2% in 8 patients (Fig. 5.3.). These occurred 16–20 h following the beginning of the infusion. Maximal prilocaine plasma levels were reached after 6–8 h [16].

5.5 Local Anesthetic Toxicity in TLA

In TLA, systemic LA toxicity occurs usually at total doses that are significantly higher than those administered using conventional local anesthetic techniques. It is likely that this results primarily from of the pharmacokinetic profile of this form of administration (see Chap. 4). Despite the high doses administered and the extensive use of the technique, there are only few reports in the medical literature on cases of local anesthetic toxicity in TLA. Klein and Kassarjdian [11] reported on one case of putative lidocaine toxicity in a patient who received 58 mg/kg of lidocaine for liposuction of the inner thighs, knees, and buttocks. Ten hours after completion of the lidocaine infusion, the patient developed nausea, vomiting, confusion, dysarthria, and ataxia. This was associated with a lidocaine plasma concentration of 6.1 mg/l (μg/ml). Perioperatively, the patient had received sertaline and flurazepam, both of which have the potential to inhibit the CYP3A4 isoenzyme of the P-450 complex and hence, lidocaine metabolism (see Sect. 4.2.3). Consequently, the authors recommended the discontinuation of drugs that potentially interfere with lidocaine metabolism at least two weeks prior to administering TLA. More recently, Rao et al. [14] reported on five deaths associated with tumescent liposuction, of which two may be linked to systemic lidocaine toxicity. However, at least two of the five patients received additional general anesthesia. The incidence of unreported cases of LA toxicity in TLA remains speculative. It should also be kept in mind that vasoconstrictor additives, although generally reducing systemic LA toxicity, carry their own potential for precipitating toxic reactions as a result of systemic absorption (Sect. 4.2.4), particularly in patients with pre-existing cardiovascular disease. Epinephrine, for example, increases the cardiovascular and CNS toxicity of bupivacaine in rats and pigs [2, 9]. Nonetheless, the practical experience with TLA indicates that the majority of patients tolerates the tumescent technique without significant problems. Toxic LA reactions can usually be controlled well in healthy patients without cardiovascular disease. This is particularly the case for the methemoglobin formation associated with prilocaine (Sect. 5.4).

5.6 Conclusion

To date, no data from prospective randomized controlled trials with sufficiently large sample sizes exist on the incidence of toxic reactions to LAs in TLA. According to the data presently available, the maximum safe dose for TLA of 55 mg/kg lidocaine recommended by the American Society for Dermatologic Surgery in 1997 [1] appears to be safe for a majority of patients. On the other hand, serious systemic toxic reactions including death may rarely occur, and careful monitoring of the patients for a sufficient length of time is crucial. Toxic reactions are potentially avoidable and often controllable, and most healthy patients without cardiovascular disease likely will tolerate TLA without significant problems.

References

1. American Society for Dermatologic Surgery (1997) Guiding principles for liposuction. Dermatol Surg 23:1127–1129
2. Bernards CM, Carpenter RL, Kenter ME, Brown DL, Rupp SM, Thompson GE (1989) Effect of epinephrine on central nervous system and cardiovascular system toxicity of bupivacaine in pigs. Anesthesiology. 71:711–7
3. Carpenter RL, Mackey DC (1992) Local anesthetics. In: Barash PG, Cullen BF, Stoelting RK (eds) Clinical anesthesia, 2nd Edition. Lippincott, Philadelphia, pp 509–541
4. Catterall WA, Mackie K (1996) Local anesthetics. In: Hardman JG, Limbird LE, Molinoff PB, Ruddon RW, Goodman Gilman A (eds) Goodman and Gilman's The pharmacological basis of therapeutics, 9th Edition. McGraw-Hill, New York, pp 331–347

5. Covino BG (1987) Toxicity and systemic effects of local anaesthetic agents. In: Strichartz GA (ed) Handbook of experimental pharmacology, vol. 81: Local anesthetics. Springer-Verlag, Berlin, pp 187–212
6. Covino BG (1988) Clinical pharmacology of local anesthetic agents. In: Cousins MJ, Bridenbaugh PO (eds) Neural blockade in clinical anesthesia and management of pain, 2nd Editon. Lippincott, Philadelphia, pp 111–144
7. de Jong RH (1994) Local anesthetics. Mosby, St. Louis
8. Hjelm M, Holmdahl MH (1965) Methemoglobinemia following lignocaine. Lancet 1:53–54
9. Kambam JR, Kinney WW, Matsuda F, Wright W, Holaday DA (1990) Epinephrine and phenylephrine increase cardiorespiratory toxicity of intravenously administered bupivacaine in rats. Anesth Analg 70:543-5
10. Klein JA (1990) Tumescent technique for regional anesthesia permits lidocaine doses of 35 mg/kg for liposuction. J Dermatol Surg Oncol 16:248–263
11. Klein JA, Kassarjdian N (1997) Lidocaine toxicity with tumescent liposuction. A case report of probable drug interactions. Dermatol Surg 23:1169–1174
12. Kreutz RW, Kinni ME (1983) Life-threatening toxic methemoglobinemia induced by prilocaine. Oral Surg Oral Med Oral Pathol 56:480–2
13. Ostad A, Kageyama N, Moy RL (1996) Tumescent anesthesia with a lidocaine dose of 55 mg/kg is safe for liposuction. Dermatol Surg 22:921–927
14. Rao RB, Ely SF, Hoffmann RS (1999) Deaths related to liposuction. N Engl J Med 340:1471–1475
15. Reynolds F (1987) Adverse effects of local anaesthetics. Br J Anaesth 59:78–95
16. Sattler G, Rapprich S, Hagedorn M (1997) Tumeszenz-Lokalanästhesie. Untersuchungen zur Pharmakokinetik von Prilocain. Z Hautkr 72:522–525
17. Strichartz GR, Berde CB (1994) Local anesthetics. In: Miller RD (ed) Anesthesia, 4th Edition. Churchill Livingstone, New York, pp 489–521
18. Tucker GT, Mather LE (1975) Pharmacology of local anaesthetic agents. Pharmacokinetics of local anaesthetic agents. Br J Anaesth 47:213–224
19. Tucker GT, Mather LE (1988) Properties, absorption, and disposition of local anesthetic agents. In: Cousins MJ, Bridenbaugh PO (eds) Neural blockade in clinical anesthesia and management of pain. Lippincott, Philadelphia, pp 47–110

6   Sedation and Analgesia

D. Bergfeld, B. Sommer

The goal of every method of anesthesia should be to keep the patient as pain-free and comfortable as possible at the lowest possible risk.

TLA is a very safe method of anesthesia [4, 10]. For many patients TLA alone is sufficient for analgesia. Some patients, however, may need extra medication. This may be caused by fear of the operation, together with consequent nervousness and increased sensitivity to pain.

Other patients perceive the infiltration of TLA as uncomfortable or painful. This is strongly related to the site of anesthesia: regions of special sensitivity are the medial side of the thigh and knee, and the periumbilical and epigastric region [1, 5].

Moreover, by giving additional sedative premedication, the infiltration rate can be raised significantly without any discomfort to the patient. This saves an enormous amount of time [5].

The fewer the medications given, the lower the risk of side effects, and the more the advantages of TLA come into effect – the first technique to make it possible to perform large operations on awake and cooperative patients.

The strong positive effect on the patient of a comfortable ambience, free from fear, and the ability to keep up an ongoing conversation with the surgeon or the OR staff, is often underestimated in the literature. Experience has shown that suitable music, if possible at a metronome tempo of about 60/min, contributes to reducing patients' tension and level of pain perception – and without any side effects.

If possible, the surgeon should maintain verbal contact with the patient throughout the duration of the infiltration. Apart from providing continuous monitoring of the patient's general condition and allowing any untoward mental or physical signs to be noticed quickly, this is also an effective way of distracting patients from the unfamiliar OR surroundings, which are often experienced as quite stressful. Our own experience has shown such measures often render additional medication unnecessary.

The individual reactive agents are discussed below; their important effects and side effects are summarized in Table 6.1.

A good rule for perioperative medication is always to restrict oneself to a few drugs with whose actions and interactions one is very familiar [7]. If medications which influence the cardiovascular system are used, appropriate monitoring equipment and treatment must be available.

Table 6.1. Sedatives and analgesics

Active substance	Diazepam	Diazepam	Midazolam	Midazolam	Midazolam	Triazolam	Paracetamol	Metamizole	Tramadol	Tilidine
Trade name	Valium	Valium	Dormicum	Dormicum	Dormicum	Halcion	Ben-u-ron	Novalgin	Tramal	Valoron N
Administration route	oral	i.v. (1 vial of 2 ml=10 mg)	Oral (Dormicum 7.5 scored film-coated tablets)	I.v. (Dormicum V 5/5 ml:1 ml contains 1 mg midazolam)	I.m. (Dormicum V 5/5 ml:1 ml contains 1 mg midazolam)	Oral (Halcion mite= triazolam 0.125 mg)	Oral tablet 500–1000 mg	Oral drops (1 ml Novalgin drops contains 500 mg metamizole)	Oral (0.5 ml= 20 drops. or 4 sqts. Tramal dr. contains 50 mg tramadol)	Oral (0.72 ml= 20 drops Valoron N sol. for oral admin. contains 50 mg tilidine and 4 mg naloxone)
Dosage	5–10 mg	5–10 mg	7.5 mg	Slow and Individual I.v.dosage: start at 1 mg, then titrate upward	0.05–0.1 mg/kg BW	0.25 mg	500–1000 mg	20–40 drops (0.5–1 g)	20–40 drops	20–40 drops
Onset of effect	10–30 min	1–2 min	10–30 min	3 min	20–30 min	30 min	20 min	10–20 min	10–20 min	15 min
Duration of effect	About 15 h	Dependent on dose up to several hours	Dependent on dose 1–3 h	45–90 min	45–90 min	Dependent on dose 1–3 h	About 4 h	About 4 h	4–6 h	3–5 h
Elimination half-life	About 30 min	24–57 h	About 30 min	1.5–2.5 h	1.5–2.5 h	1.5–3 h	About 2 h	4–7 h	6 h	3 h

Drug interactions	Drop in blood pressure, especially if rapidly injected. Drop in blood pressure. Risk of acumulation. Pain along the vein, possibility of thrombophlebitis	Drop in blood pressure, especially in combination with opioids	Drop in blood pressure, especially in combination with opioids. Enhancement of effects by: ranitidine, erythromycin, diltiazem, verapamil, ketoconazole, itraconazole	Drop in blood pressure, especially in combination with opioids. Enhancement of effects by: ranitidine, erythromycin, diltiazem, verapamil, ketoconazole, itraconazole	Drop in blood pressure, especially in combination with opioids. Enhancement of effects by: ranitidine, erythromycin, diltiazem, verapamil, ketoconazole, itraconazole	Ketoconazole, itroconazole, cimetidine, verapamil, diltiazem, isoniazide, erythromycin, macrolide antibiotics	Onset of effect delayed by medications that enhance emptying of the stomach (metoclopramide)	Antihypertensives and diuretics may alter effects	Enhances effects of CNS-depressing drugs and alcohol	Enhances effects of CNS-depressing drugs and alcohol
Side effects	Respiratory depression, especially with fast injection. Drop in blood pressure. Risk of acumulation. Pain along the vein, possibility of thrombophlebitis	Respiratory depression. Benzodiazepine incompatibility	Respiratory depression, anterograde amnesia. Drop in blood pressure. Rarely, paradoxical reactions in elderly patients	Respiratory depression, anterograde amnesia. Drop in blood pressure. Rarely, paradoxical reactions in elderly patients	Respiratory depression, anterograde amnesia. Drop in blood pressure. Rarely, paradoxical reactions in elderly patients	Tachycardia, somnambulism, euphoria	Analgetic asthma in predisposed patients	Agranulocytosis extremely rarely. Kidney disorders when given long-term	Orthostatic regulation disorders, nausa	Orthostatic regulation disorders, nausea
Contradications	Myasthenia gravis. Benzodiazepine incompatibility	Myasthenia gravis. Benzodiazepine hypersensitivity	Acute narrow-angle glaucoma, known benzodiazepine hypersensitivity	Acute narrow-angle glaucoma, known benzodiazepine hypersensitivity	Acute narrow-angle glaucoma, known benzodiazepine hypersensitivity	Severe psychiatric illnesses	Liver function disorders	Bone marrow disorders. Congenital glucose-6-phosphate-dehydrogenase deficiency	Acute drug intoxication and drug substitution	Acute drug intoxication and drug substitution
Other	Antagonist: flumazenil (Anexate) initially 0.2 mg, then increase in 0.1-mg increments	Antagonist: flumazenil (Anexate) initially 0.2 mg, then increase in 0.1-mg increments	Antagonist: flumazenil (Anexate) initially 0.2 mg, then increase in 0.1-mg increments	Antagonist: flumazenil (Anexate) initially 0.2 mg, then increase in 0.1-mg increments	Antagonist: flumazenil (Anexate) initially 0.2 mg, then increase in 0.1-mg increments but	Not available in Germany as premedication, only for treatment of sleep disorders			Side effects enhanced by motion	Side effects enhanced by motion

6.1   Perioperative Sedation

The main substances used are tranquilizers, which have a calming effect and reduce excessive anxiety and tension. At the usual dosage their chief effect is on the limbic system. They reduce psychologically induced excitation of autonomic neurons, thereby uncoupling psychological and autonomic processes. At higher dosages, their general suppression of the propagation of excitatory impulses has an anticonvulsant effect. Interactions with substances in the TLA solution are not to be expected, so the usual dose recommendations, contraindications, and drug interactions apply.

6.1.1   Benzodiazepines

The many benzodiazepines currently available on the market have very similar ranges of effects: anxiolytic, sedative-hypnotic, muscle relaxant, and anticonvulsant [13]. They are especially suited as premedications in regional anesthesia because they have a protective effect against cerebral seizures, which are promoted by local anesthetic.

Contraindications for all benzodiazepines include: acute narrow-angle glaucoma, severe liver damage, and pulmonary function disorders, e.g., chronic bronchitis or bronchial asthma.

The most common side effects are drowsiness and decreased reactivity. This should be explained to patients prior to outpatient procedures, so that the matter of escorts and transport home can be discussed in good time. Other dangerous side effects such as a drop in blood pressure or respiratory depression are rare at the dosages given, but should always be ruled out by appropriate monitoring.

The effects of centrally acting pharmaceuticals and analgesics may be enhanced. In particular, the slight cardiovascular effects observed when the benzodiazepines are given alone may be increased when they are combined with opioids [6].

Diazepam (e.g., Valium)

Diazepam is one of the longest-acting benzodiazepines. It can be administered orally at a dose of 5–10 mg on the evening before the procedure to give the patient a good night's sleep.

Perioperatively, it can also be given orally at the same dose [8]. Oral administration is safer and longer-lasting than parenteral administration [7]. Onset of effect is after about 10–30 min.

When administering diazepam intravenously it is usual to give an initial dose of 5 mg, and then to add another 5 mg if the results are insufficient. Side effects of intravenous administration are pain along the course of the vein and, sometimes, thrombophlebitis, caused by the binder propylene glycol.

Midazolam (Dormicum)

Before major procedures, midazolam can be given as premedication at a dosage of 0.05–0.1 mg/kg body weight i.m. 20–30 min before the operation. Some American authors recommend a standard dose of 5 mg i.m. [5].

If administered intravenously, an initial dose of 1 mg should be given slowly. If sedation is inadequate, the same dose can be repeated after at least 2 min.

Because the individual pharmacodynamics vary enormously with midazolam, carefully titration of doses is recommended until the desired degree of sedation is reached [2,11]. Higher doses should only be given if respiration and circulation can be monitored. In healthy patients below the age of 60 years, a maximum dose of 5.0 mg should not be exceeded. In patients over 60 years of age or those with cardiorespiratory diseases, especially chronic obstructive lung conditions, severe CNS disease, or liver function deficits, a maximum dose of 3.5 mg should not be exceeded.

After the administration of midazolam, patient reactivity will be considerably decreased. Patients should be discharged no earlier than 3 h after receiving the drug, and then only with an escort.

Midazolam injection solution should not be used in patients with schizophrenia or endogenous depression, because there is a risk of acute exacerbation.

Midazolam is one of the short-acting benzodiazepines, and may therefore be considered as very safe. Repeat injections may be needed in protracted procedures [7,11].

Triazolam (Halcion)

In Germany, triazolam is not routinely used for perioperative sedation, but it is used by American surgeons. The recommended oral dose is 0.25 mg on the evening before the procedure and 1 h preoperatively. It can cause slight perioperative amnesia – which may well be seen as desirable [8].

6.1.2 Neuroleptics

Psychomotor excitations are reduced by neuroleptics, which are sedative and depress the autonomic nervous system. Only at dosages above the neuroleptic threshold does their antipsychotic action in schizophrenic or psychotic patients start to take effect.

Neuroleptics are divided into the mild and the potent. Mild neuroleptics are preferred in outpatient procedures, partly because of their antihistaminic, antiemetic, and analgesic side effects.

The main contraindications are severe liver and kidney function disorders, pre-existing cardiac conditions, and chronic lung disease.

Side effects can be caused by the anticholinergic effects of the substance (e.g., micturition disorders, constipation, accommodation disturbances, tachycardia). In rare cases, dyskinesia and orthostatic disregulation have also been reported.

Drugs with centrally calming effects enhance the action of neuroleptics, caffeine reduces it.

Promethazine (Atosil)

Promethazine is a neuroleptic of the phenothiazine type. A dose of 12.5–25 mg i.m. is suitable for anesthesia premedication. In addition to its sedative effects, promethazine also has antiemetic properties and acts as an antihistamine [3].

Dose recommendation: 25 mg i.m. about 30 min before the beginning of the injection [8].

Triflupromazine (Psyquil)

Triflupromazine can be used perioperatively for tranquilization in a dose of 20 mg i.m. or 5–10 mg i.v.

Occasionally, in patients with a relevant history, reactivation of psychotic processes may occur.

Clonidine

Arterial hypertonia is the main indication for the α_2-adrenoreceptor agonist clonidine. Because it has a strong sedative effect without affecting respiration, it is recommended by Jeff Klein, the "originator" of the tumescent technique, as a potent additional medication in procedures using local anesthesia [7].

Clonidine has a distinct analgesic effect and can enhance the effects of benzodiazepines. Also, it has a negative chronotropic effect. This sometimes can be desirable when tachycardias occur, e.g., in liposuction with TLA. In patients with pre-existing bradycardiac arrhythmias, however, continual monitoring of the heart rate is essential if clonidine is given.

The drop in blood pressure triggered by clonidine is normally clinically insignificant when the drug is carefully given in small doses; indeed, it may even help prevent postoperative bleeding [9].

The oral dose recommended by Klein is 0.1 mg just prior to the procedure. In the German-speaking countries, this additional medication has not yet been introduced.

6.2   Perioperative Analgesia

Not much experience has been gained pre- or postoperatively with additional use of peripheral or central analgesics in TLA.

The use of additional analgesics may be worthwhile during infiltration in especially painful areas (as mentioned above). However, it should be re-emphasized that this is not routinely necessary, since most patients tolerate the injection without any problems.

When the administration of an additional analgesic is considered, it is a good idea to give only a peripheral, nonopioid preparation, or to combine a peripheral and a central analgesic, in order to profit from the different sites of action of these preparations and to keep their respective side effects as low as possible by keeping the dosage low. Such combinations are routinely used to induce anesthesia and are presented below.

If increased pain sensitivity is antici-pated even before the procedure starts, the medication should be given in good time (about 0.5–1 h) before the operation.

If the patient is also to be sedated, the possibility of additive central effects should be taken into account when using central analgesics.

6.2.1 Peripheral Analgesics

For preference, nonacidic antipyretic analgesics (pyrazole derivatives) such as paracetamol and metamizole are used. At normal therapeutic dosage, the undesirable adverse effects of this preparation group can be regarded as relatively mild [12]. Drug interactions are also rare. The pyrazolones probably act at the spinal level by influencing nociceptive afferences on the caudal horn. Whether they also influence the prostaglandin metabolism like other peripheral analgesics is not known, but the antiphlogistic effect is very slight.

Contraindications for higher doses are severe liver and kidney function disorders.

Paracetamol

In a single dose of 500–1000 mg, paracetamol is generally well tolerated preoperatively and has few side effects. If necessary, paracetamol can also be used to treat postoperative pain.

The maximum daily dose should not exceed 3000 mg.

Metamizole

In the form of drops metamizole is especially suited for combination with a central analgesic.

The recommended dose is 15–20 (–40) drops postoperatively.

Parenteral administration can lead to an acute drop in blood pressure and may only be used when facilities for shock treatment are available. Possible side effects are hypersensitive reactions, e.g., in the skin and mucous membranes. The most severe adverse reaction, agranulocytosis, mostly occurs when the drug is given at high doses and over long periods, but overall it is very rare.

6.2.2 Central Analgesics

Mild opioid analgesics with some antagonistic effects are used perioperatively. Only in exceptional cases is there a need for more potent preparations that are controlled substances and have more extensive adverse effects.

Opioid analgesics also have an entirely desirable psychological sedative effect.

Dangerous side effects are not expected in these mild preparations. Possible respiratory depression should be watched for, although it is less pronounced in a patient in acute pain. Nevertheless, it should be borne in mind, especially when mild opioid analgesics are used in combination with sedatives and in patients with obstructive respiratory disease. Perioperatively, the hypostatic and emetogenic effects of these drugs should also be remembered. The respiratory depressive effect can last significantly longer than the analgesia, requiring continued observation [7].

Since these effects are enhanced by movement, it is better to get the patient changed, etc., before administering the opioid analgesic.

Contraindications are a hypertrophic prostate, bile duct diseases, disorders of respiratory function, and an increased tendency to cerebral seizures.

Mild opioids

Tramadol (e.g., Tramal)
Tramadol is supplied in different forms (capsules, tablets, suppositories, drops, injectable solution). The potency is about one-quarter that of morphine. The single dose for healthy adults is 50–100 mg postoperatively.

In drop form, the dose is 15–20 (-40) postoperatively.

Tilidine and naloxone (Valoron)
Tilidine and naloxone as a fixed combination in Valoron are generally given in the form of drops. The single dose is 50–100 mg postoperatively, which equals 20–40 drops.

Potent opioids

As mentioned above, potent opioids are needed only in exceptional cases and require monitoring and continued observation of the patient because of the possible adverse effects. Respiratory depression is the most serious adverse effect. The respiratory depression lasts longer than the analgesic effect (protracted respiratory depression). Giving tranquilizers at the same time can enhance the central-acting side effects. For this reason they should be employed with caution in outpatients.

Piritramide (Dipidolor)
Piritramide is a little less potent than morphine, but lasts significantly longer (about 6 h).

For severe pain, piritramide can be given intramuscularly, subcutaneously, or intravenously. When given subcutaneously or intramuscularly, the individual dose is 15–30 mg; when given intravenously it must be injected slowly (10 mg/min). Elderly patients and patients in a poor general condition of health or with liver function disorders should be given smaller doses.

Pethidine (Meperidin)
Pethidine is used by American surgeons in procedures in TLA. The recommended dose is 25–100 mg i.v. or i.m. Generally, 50 mg is given intramuscularly [7,5].

One thing to remember is that pethidine can lead to hypotension and tachycardia more often than other opioids [3].

Fentanyl

Since the introduction of neuroleptic analgesia, fentanyl has been one of the most important analgesics in anesthesia. It is about 100 times more potent than morphine. The duration of effect is 30 min.

For cosmetic procedures, the recommended dose is 0.5–2.0 µg/kg given parenterally [7].

Experience with our own patients has shown that to use such a potent preparation is unnecessary in TLA.

The long-acting analgesic effects of TLA usually make further postoperative pain medication unnecessary (see Chap. 4). If required, a peripheral analgesic with few side effects, e.g., paracetamol, is generally given.

For more severe pain, tramadol has shown good analgesic effects in the postoperative period without causing constipation and micturition disturbances as morphine does [6].

References

1. Coleman WP, Letessier S, Hanke CW (1997) Liposuction. In: Coleman WP III, Hanke CW, Alt TH, Asken S (eds) Cosmetic surgery of the skin. 2nd Edition, Mosby, pp 178–206
2. Diem E (1989) Kontrollierte Analgosedierung zur Erleichterung ausgedehnter Eingriffe in Lokalanästhesie. In: Fortschritte der operativen Dermatologie, vol 5. Breuninger H (eds) Operationsplanung und Erfolgskontrolle, Springer, Berlin Heidelberg New York Tokyo, pp 43–46
3. Doenicke A (1995) Pharmaka für die Prämedikation. In: Doenicke A, Kettler D, List WF, Radke J, Tarnow J (eds), Anästhesiologie, 7th edn. Springer, Berlin Heidelberg New York Tokyo, pp 35–55
4. Hanke CW, Bernstein G, Bullock BS (1995) Safety of tumescent liposuction in 15,336 patients – national survey results. Dermatol Surg 21:459–462
5. Hanke CW, Coleman WP et al. (1997) Infusion rates and levels of premedication in tumescent liposuction. Dermatol Surg 23:1131–1134
6. Hoeft A, Kettler D (1995) Interaktion von Anästhetika und anderen Pharmaka. In: Doenicke A, Kettler D, List WF, Radke J, Tarnow J (eds), Anästhesiologie, 7th edn. Springer, Berlin Heidelberg New York Tokyo, S. 319–324
7. Klein J (1997) Anesthesia for dermatologic cosmetic surgery. In: Coleman WP III, Hanke CW, Alt TH, Asken S (eds) Cosmetic surgery of the skin, 2nd edn, Mosby, pp 62–71
8. Narins RS, Coleman WP III (1997) Minimizing pain for liposuction anesthesia. Dermatol Surg 23:1137–1140
9. Singelyn FJ, Gouverneur JM, Robert A (1996) A minimum dose of clonidine added to mepivacaine prolongs the duration of anesthesia and analgesia after axillary brachial plexus block. Anesth Analg (1996) 83:1046–1050
10. The American Academy of Cosmetic Surgery (1997) Guidelines for liposuction surgery. Am J Cosm 14:389–393
11. Wresch KP (1995) Analgosedierung zur Supplementierung der inkompletten Regionalanästhesie. Anasthesist 44:580–587
12. Zenz M, Jurna I (1993) Lehrbuch der Schmerztherapie. Wissenschaftliche Verlagsgesellschaft, Stuttgart
13. Zoebe A (1988) Praeoperative Sedierung. In: Haneke E (ed) Gegenwärtiger Stand der operativen Dermatologie. Fortschritte der operativen Dermatologie, vol 4. Springer, Berlin Heidelberg, pp 47–50

7   Prevention of Infection and Thrombosis

D. BERGFELD, B. SOMMER

7.1   Perioperative Infection Prophylaxis

There is some controversy as to whether perioperative infection prophylaxis is routinely necessary or not [8]. In general and in small procedures on the cutis, antibiotic prophylaxis is not indicated [2]. Because of the bacteriostatic effect of the local anesthetic and the wash-out effect of the TLA solution mentioned earlier (see Chap. 8), the risk of infection is very slim in procedures performed under TLA anyway. Nevertheless, many surgeons like to provide additional antibiotic protection for the patient, especially in extended operations such as liposuction or surgery for varicose veins.

A short course or a single administration prior to the operation is recommended. The antibiotics should protect especially against staphylococci, or, if possible, also against other microorganisms.

For perioperative prophylaxis in liposuction procedures in our patients we have had good experiences with the gyrase inhibitor ciprofloxacin given postoperatively as 250 mg twice daily over a period of 3 days, starting on the day of surgery.

Another suitable antibiotic is cephuroximatexil (Elobact or Zinnat) 250 mg twice daily[2].

The perioperative single-shot administration of, e.g., 200 mg ciprofloxacin i.v. protects effectively against postoperative complications in surgery on the venous system [7]. Also suitable is cefotiam (Spizef) 1 g [2].

If signs of an infection occur despite ongoing antibiotic prophylaxis, blood cultures should be performed or a swab taken from the wound to identify the pathogen before the antibiotic is changed [1].

7.2   Perioperative Thrombosis Prophylaxis

Since TLA is a method of local anesthesia, making immediate postoperative mobilization of the patients possible, no routine antithrombosis medication such as heparin treatment is necessary. In addition, the tumescent solution has been postulated to have an antithrombotic effect (see Chap. 4). For high-risk patients, major procedures, or extended operative time (> 45 min) antithrombotic medication may be indicated and is then given at the usual dosage [4, 5] (Tables 7.1, 7.2).

Physical measures are recommended in all thrombosis risk categories. The effectiveness of thrombosis prophylaxis stockings has long been proven [6]; nevertheless, some points still need to be taken into account here. The usual white

Table 7.1. Categories of thrombosis risk adapted from Partsch and Blättler [4] and Nicolaides et al. [3]

Risk category	Nature of surgery	Prophylaxis
High	Major[a] surgery, age > 60 Major surgery, age 40–60, with malignant tumor or history of thromboembolism Thrombophilia	Physical thrombosis prophylaxis (antithrombosis stockings) Low-molecular-weight heparin in the recommended dose for high-risk patients (4000–5000 anti-FXa-units every 24 h) Oral anticoagulants Standard heparin 5000 units twice daily
Intermediate	Major surgery, age 40–50, without other risk factors Minor[b] surgery, age > 60 Minor surgery, age 40–60, with history of thromboembolism or estrogen therapy	Physical thrombosis prophylaxis (antithrombosis stockings) Low-molecular-weight heparin (2000–3000 units anti-FXa-units or standard heparin 5000 units twice daily
Low	Major surgery, age <40 without other risk factors Minor surgery, age 40–60, with no risk factors	Physical thrombosis prophylaxis (antithrombosis stockings)

[a] Major surgery: duration of op. (or op. time) over 45 min
[b] Minor surgery: duration of op. (or op. tim) under 45 min [3]

Table 7.2. Predisposing risk factors for thromboembolism [5]

1. Congenital risk factors	2. Acquired risk factors
APC (activated protein C) resistency	Lupus anticoagulant and antiphospholipid
Antithrombin-III-deficiency	antibodies, nephrotic syndrome, paroxysmal
Protein C-deficiency	nocturnal hemoglobinuria, malignant tumors,
Dysfibrinogenemia	cardiac insufficiency, advanced age, estrogen
Fibrinolysis disturbances	therapy, sepsis, immobilization, stroke,
Homocysteinemia	polycythemia, inflammatory bowel disease, obesity, varicosis, previous thromboembolisms

thigh-length antithrombosis stockings have the disadvantage that they almost constantly slip down, forming a crease in the popliteal region and restricting the lower circulation. The edema of the lower leg occasionally seen as a result has led many clinicians to rename them "thrombosis stockings." The problem can be prevented by prescribing knee-length stockings instead, since it is in the lower leg that most of the venous pooling takes place.

Our department has had good experiences with a special compression bandage stocking, which is individually fitted and does not normally crease (Struva

35 or 23, medi Bayreuth Co.; see Appendix C). Depending on the model, this stocking provides 23 or 35 mmHg in the ankle area, a defined continuous pressure gradient between compression classes 2 and 3, and a practical suspending system at the thigh to prevent slippage (see Chap. 28). Their clinical effectiveness has now been demonstrated [9].

With *heparin*, the *contraindications* must be respected. Absolute contraindications are known cerebral aneurysm, aortic aneurysm, or an aortic dissection. Relative contraindications are simultaneous treatment with nonsteroidal anti-inflammatory drugs, platelet function inhibitors, or valproic acid (antiepileptic drugs).

Another factor to remember when weighing up the pros and cons of thromboembolism prophylaxis with heparin is the rare risk of *heparin-induced thrombopenia*. Therefore, it is currently recommended to monitor thrombocytes once or twice a week before beginning prophylaxis. Thromboses and occlusion of blood vessels can occur in heparin-induced type II thrombopenia, which is caused immunologically by the formation of heparin antibodies ("white clot syndrome").

References

1. Coleman WP, Letessier S, Hanke CW (1997) Liposuction. In: Coleman WP III, Hanke CW, Alt TH, Asken S (eds) Cosmetic surgery of the skin, 2nd edn. Mosby, St Louis
2. Gloor S, Ringelmann R (1996) Antibiotika in der Dermatologie. Z Hautkr 71:672–677
3. Nicolaides AN, Bergqvist R (1995) Prevention of venous thromboembolism. International consensus statement under the auspices of the cardiovascular disease education and research trust and the International Union of Angiology. London, 7th April 1995
4. Partsch H, Blaettler W (1996) Leitlinien zur Thrombose-Prophylaxe. Phlebol 25:261–266
5. Partsch H, Blaettler W, Hertel T (1998) Leitlinien zur Thromboseprophylaxe. Gemeinsam verabschiedete Leitlinien der deutschen Gesellschaft für Phlebologie und der gemeinsamen Qualitätssicherungskommission der Deutschen Dermatologischen Gesellschaft und des Berufsverbandes der Deutschen Dermatologen e.V., Juli 1997. D.T. derm: 46, Heft 1
6. Partsch H, Kahn P (1982) Venöse Strömungsbeschleunigung in Bein und Becken durch „Anti-Thombose-Strümpfe". Klinikarzt 11:609–615
7. Salzmann G, Kirschner P, Hoffmann O, Vanderpuy R (1995) Perioperative Antibiotikaprophylaxe bei der paratibialen Fasziotomie. Phlebol 24:44–47
8. The American Academy of Cosmetic Surgery (1997) Guidelines for liposuction surgery. Am J Cosm Surg 14:389–393
9. Wrobel R, Gussmann A, Dahse HP, Metz L (1996) Messung des Kompressionseffektes von Kompressionsbinden und Strumpfverbänden. Vortrag im Rahmen der 38. Tagung der Deutschen Gesellschaft für Phlebologie, Berlin, 25–29 September 1996

8   Advantages and Disadvantages of TLA

B. SOMMER

8.1   Specific Advantages of TLA

The specific advantages of TLA are summarized in the following list and are discussed in detail later on.
- Complete anesthesia of large areas
- Hydrodissection as a surgical tool
- Less bleeding = fewer hematomas
- Improved hematoma resorption = less postoperative pain
- Safe method compared to local anesthetic and intubation anesthesia
- Protracted effect of the local anesthetic = less postoperative pain
- Antibacterial action of TLA solution
- Antibacterial effect from wash-out effect of TLA solution
- Compensation of intraoperative fluid loss

8.1.1   Size of the Anesthetized Area

The tumescent technique has revolutionized traditional methods of local anesthesia. Because the anesthetic solution used in TLA is so dilute and high doses of local anesthetic can be administered with safety, even very large areas of the body can be anesthetized.

Liposuction is the procedure which requires the largest amount of local anesthetic compared to other procedures in surgical dermatology. This is because of the need to achieve adequate anesthesia of the entire subcutaneous fatty tissue, which varies from individual to individual. In procedures that only require anesthesia of the surface skin layers, less TLA solution can be used.

8.1.2   Safety

The extraordinary safety of this method was demonstrated by an impressive questionnaire-based survey by the American Society for Dermatologic Surgery that evaluated data on 15,336 patients who underwent liposuction under TLA according to the guidelines [1,2]. Complications were very rare. Table 8.1. gives an overview of the findings.

Table 8.1. Complications in 15,336 patients with liposuction under tumescent local anesthesia (adapted from [1])

Complication	Number of patients	%
Infection	52	0.3391
Postoperative focal, subcutaneous, panniculitis-like reaction	30	0.1956
Hematomas/seromas	26	0.1695
Allergic reaction to additional medication or adhesive tape	18	0.1174
Persistent postoperative edema	15	0.0978
Nausea not associated with other analgesics	11	0.0717
Vasovagal reaction or syncope	11	0.0717
Excessive or persistent postoperative pain	9	0.0587
Postoperative fever	8	0.0522
Abnormally extended ecchymoses	5	0.0362
Unusual postoperative sleepiness/tiredness	5	0.0362
Permanent damage of sensitive nerves	5	0.0362
Cardiac arrhythmias requiring therapy	0	0
Anemia	0	0
Complications resulting in hospitalization	0	0
Blood or fluid losses requiring transfusions	0	0
Venous or fat embolism	0	0
Hypovolemic shock	0	0
Perforation of peritoneum or thorax	0	0
Seizures	0	0
Thrombophlebitis	0	0
Toxic reactions to intravenous sedative or narcotic	0	0
Death	0	0

8.1.3 Hydrodissection

The high interstitial pressure caused by the infiltrated volumes effects pre-preparation of the subcutaneous tissue along the existing connective tissue structures. This advantage can be used as a surgical "tool" in:
- Skin flaps; to facilitate the mobilization (see Chap. 18)
- Vein surgery, since mobilization is along the beds of the veins (see Chap. 28)
- Liposuction; to stretch the connective tissue fibers and loosen the adhesion of adiposities from the connective tissue (see Chap. 12)

8.1.4 Hemostasis

The high tissue pressure after the infiltration and the addition of vasoconstrictors results in decreased circulation at the surgical site. This helps prevent the formation of large hematomas. At the same time, blood transfusions become unnecessary in liposuction procedures, unlike the case with out-dated "dry" liposuction techniques.

8.1.5 Analgesic Effects

The slow infiltration rate of TLA and the extreme lipophilia of the local anesthetic together with the added vasoconstrictors causes a protracted duration of effect which often renders postoperative pain medication unnecessary.

8.1.6 Postoperative Complications

If hematomas occur (which cannot always be prevented in extended liposuction procedures and long operations on the venous system), they are much more easily resorbed because of the diluting effect of the large volumes of tumescent solution still remaining in the tissue. Also, the antibacterial effect of the local anesthetic together with the wash-out effect of the TLA solution draining from the skin incisions acts against infection. These facts explain the clinical observation that hematoma and complication rates are noted less often than in vein surgery under general anesthesia. No data from controlled studies are yet available. In addition, the decreased risk of thrombosis helps to minimize the rate of postoperative complications.

8.1.7 Intraoperative Fluid Loss

The large volume of subcutaneously infiltrated isotonic saline or Ringer´s solution acts like an interstitial infusion. Therefore, there is no need to replace intraoperative fluid loss by intravenous infusion. Resorbed carrier solution is excreted by the kidney without complications. In addition, the unnecessary intravenous fluid infusion could promote the formation of pulmonary edema in patients with compensated cardiac insufficiency.

8.1.8 Comparison of Tumescent Anesthesia and General Anesthesia

For extended dermatological surgery that will require general anesthesia if TLA is not possible, the advantages and disadvantages of each method should be considered. A comparison of TLA and intubation anesthesia gives the following:
Advantages of TLA in comparison to general anesthesia
- Fewer perioperative diagnostic procedures necessary.
- Even patients who are high-risk in relation to intubation anesthesia can be operated.
- The anesthesiologist need only be on call.
- Great intraoperative safety.
- Fewer hematomas.

- Long-lasting pain relief.
- Patient can change position him/herself during the operation.
- Postoperative mobilization is ideal.
- Shorter hospital stay or outpatient procedure.
- Cost savings.

8.2 Specific Disadvantages of TLA

Specific disadvantages of TLA are summarized below:
- TLA fluid in the surgical site.
- Infiltration is time-consuming.
- Inadequate sedation is a potential stress for surgeon and patient.
- Patient needs to be communicated with throughout the procedure.
- Assessment of the anesthetized surgical site is more difficult.
- It can be difficult to identify sources of bleeding.

8.2.1 TLA Fluid in the Surgical Site

The great volume of fluid results in a "dripping wet" surgical site in varicose vein surgery that takes getting used to. Because of the high tissue pressure, the lumina of the blood vessels seem smaller than suggested by the perioperative diagnostic procedures [3]. On the other hand, varicose veins, for example, are in effect "pre-prepared" by the accumulation of fluid in the perivascular space. This is an especially useful effect in phlebectomy and prevents postoperative hematomas, pain, and risk of infection.

8.2.2 Infiltration Time

Depending on the procedure, the infiltration of large areas consumes varying lengths of time. For the infiltration of a junction of the small saphenous vein one needs about 3–5 min, whereas anesthesia for extensive liposuction of the hip and thighs can take up to 1.5 h.

8.2.3 Disadvantages Due to Insufficient Sedation

In principle, TLA can be carried out without any sedation. Depending on the patient and the planned duration of the procedure, however, the lack of adequate sedation can lead to nervousness, especially when intraoperative complications occur. As in all procedures under local anesthesia, the surgeon, assistant, and OR nurse can have only limited communication during the procedure in order not to worry the patient. If an operation takes longer than expected, this can also cause psychological and physical strain because the patient must lie in an uncomfortable position for a long time.

8.2.4 Patient Management During Surgery

Extended operations lasting several hours require extra attentiveness by the surgeon because he or she must concentrate simultaneously on the surgery and on the awake patient. Relaxing music played at a comfortable volume and an even tempo (metronome setting) has proven very helpful in calming the patient. Equally helpful is music provided by the patient him-/herself, so long as the OR staff can also live with it.

8.2.5 Changes in Skin Relief

Because of the large volumes, the skin tension lines smooth out and the whole surgical site swells up (*tumescere*=to swell) and becomes unrecognizable. Therefore, precise preoperative marking is particularly important in this method of anesthesia, since there should be no "change of direction" during surgery. In cancer surgery, tumor borders become unrecognizable, in liposuctions other areas that might also require treatment can no longer be identified, and in skin flap procedures the esthetic units merge, making precise operative planning at this stage impossible.

8.2.6 Identifying Sources of Bleeding

The search for potential postoperative sources of bleeding can be made more difficult by the tissue compression and the added epinephrine. Especially in extended operations in acne inversa, meticulous intraoperative hemostasis is essential, since the lack of compressibility of the surgical site means that even small vessel bleeds may lead to revision surgery.

References

1. Hanke CW, Bernstein G, Bullock BS (1995) Safety of tumescent liposuction in 15,336 patients-national survey results. Dermatol Surg 21:459–462
2. Hanke CW, Bullock BS, Bernstein G (1996) Current status of tumescent liposuction in the United States, national survey results. Dermatol Surg 22:595–598
3. Jokisch R, Sattler G, Hagedorn M (1998) Vena saphena parva-Resektion in Tumeszenz-lokalanästhesie. phlebologie 27:48–50

Part B

Practical Application

9   Infiltration Technique

D. BERGFELD, B. SOMMER, G. SATTLER

Before the start of TLA, the skin in the area to be anesthetized is disinfected with one of the common preparations.

In general, it is advisable to primarily make small subcutaneous wheals with a local anesthetic at normal concentration; cannulas can then be painlessly inserted into these and the TLA solution infiltrated into the surrounding tissue in a fan-shaped pattern.

TLA can of course be injected with any kind of syringe or cannula, like any other local anesthetic. To reach the largest possible area with one injection, however, long injection cannulas should be used, e.g., a conventional single-use cannula 0.9 mm in diameter and 4–7 cm (1.5–2.5 inches) in length. Since the treated area is generally so large that the syringe would have to be refilled several times, this infiltration technique is only suitable for small cases.

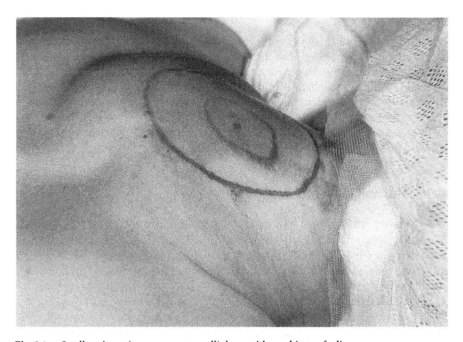

Fig. 9.1.   Swollen tissue (*tumescere*=to swell), here with markings of a lipoma

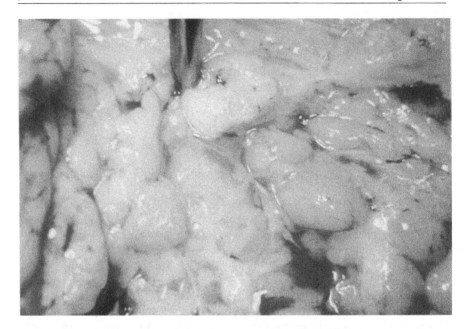

Fig. 9.2. Complete saturation of the subcutaneous fat with TLA solution, demonstrated intraoperatively. Typical of tumescence are the bloodlessness of the surgical site and the red-tinged fluid accumulations, due to dilution of leaking blood by TLA solution

During the infiltration, the skin turgor is monitored by constant palpation, and verbal contact is continued with the patient in order to monitor the level of consciousness. The infiltration is complete when a bulging, elastic skin turgor (*tumescere*= to swell) is reached. The infiltrated area can be easily distinguished because of the swelling and the blanching effect of the epinephrine; exploratory percussion will reveal an almost watermelon-like consistency (Fig. 9.1).

In extended excisions, the complete saturation of the subcutaneous fat with TLA solution can also be demonstrated intraoperatively (Fig. 9.2).

9.1   Manual Infiltration

Percutaneous sticks, which deliver the TLA solution from larger infusion bags, were developed relatively early for manual infiltration. This technique of manual infiltration is still used for anesthesia of limited surgical sites. The percutaneous sticks are manufactured with 2- to 10-ml piston stroke (reusable syringes by, e.g., Nechmad Intl., Israel; Wells Johnson Co., USA; or 10-ml disposable syringes by Byron Medical, USA; see Appendix C) (Figs. 9.3–9.5).

These syringes aspirate the TLA solution with each stroke via a normal infusion set, e.g., from a 500-ml bag on an infusion stand, and inject it into the tissue with the next stroke. The advantages of this technique are: more precise infiltra-

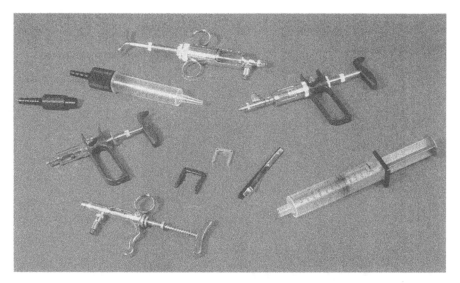

Fig. 9.3. Various percutaneous sticks by different manufacturers: Wells Johnson (*back*) and Nechmad (*front*) (see Appendix C)

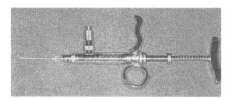

Fig. 9.4. Example of a sterilizable percutaneous stick (Wells Johnson and Nechmad)

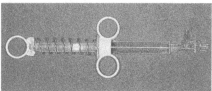

Fig. 9.5. Example of a disposable percutaneous stick (Byron Medical)

tion, easy adjustability of the infiltration rate, and minimal risk of inadvertent intravascular infiltration, because volume per piston stroke is restricted. Disadvantages include: a significant physical strain in extensive procedures and a low maximum infiltration rate.

9.2 Mechanical Infiltration

Where large volumes of TLA are needed, e.g., when 6 l dilute solution are injected, electrically powered automatic pump systems are more efficient.

Jeffrey Klein, the originator of TLA, developed a roll pump system which is available through HK Surgical (Adress see part C). The volume delivered per minute by this pump can be adjusted, thus varying the infiltration rate.

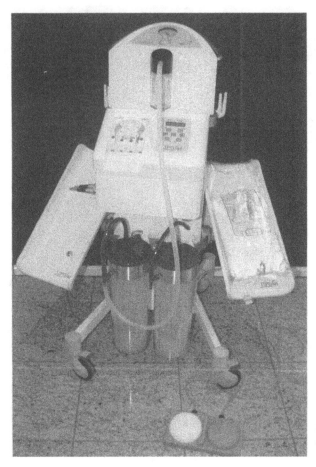

Fig. 9.6. Sophisticated Mechanical roll pump: „LipoSat" (LaserPoint)

The latest pump ("LipoSat") can deliver between 40 and 200 ml/min. The infiltration cannulas are available with one or more holes in the needle through which the TLA solution "pours" into the subcutaneous fat as from a watering can. Standard diameters are 1.5, 2.0, and 3 mm, with lengths varying from 10 to 40 cm. Such infiltration needles are especially useful in the anesthesia of deeper layers of fatty tissue, e.g., in abdominal liposuction.

The pump manufactured by LaserPoint (Adress see part C; Fig. 9.6) has many unique features: The solution is warmed up, the flow volume is measured electronically, the infiltration volume can be pre-selected.

A number of other systems now also exist, available from LaserPoint in Germany or from manufacturers in Argentina (Figs. 9.7 and 9.8, see Appendix C).

With each of these pump systems, the physician ensures that the TLA solution is pumped into the tissue at a number of injection sites, spreading out in a fan shape from each, thus ensuring optimal distribution of the TLA solution and even tumescence. The duration of the infiltration depends on the infiltration rate and may be more than 1 h when large volumes of TLA are being used, especially since too high an infiltration rate causes a rapid buildup of pressure that may be uncomfortable for the patient. Too rapid infiltration also has other disadvantages (see Sect. 4.5). All this gave rise to the idea of shortening the infiltration procedure by using several injection cannulas at the same time, delivering the

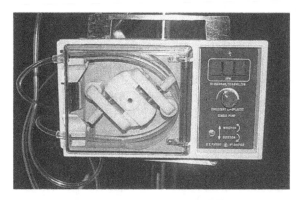

Fig. 9.7. Mechanical roll pump: Blugerman pump (Shavelzon)

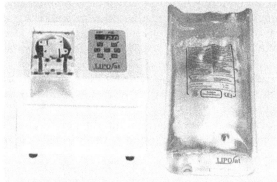

Fig. 9.8. Electronic roll pump system according to Dr. Sattler, including a warming dish for the tumescence Solution (LaserPoint)

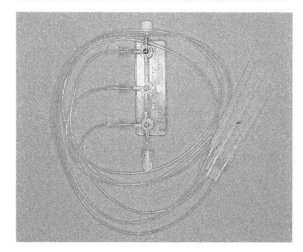

Fig. 9.9. Sattler distributor (LaserPoint)

fluid relatively slowly from each individual cannula. Distribution of the solution to the various tubes is facilitated by a combination of ordinary three-way stopcocks, or, alternatively, by the Sattler distributor recently developed especially for TLA (Intra, Germany) (Fig. 9.9). Here, one infusion system supplies three or six needles which distribute the solution at different locations in the surgical site.

9.3 Temporal Dynamics of Infiltration

For successful TLA, it is essential to consider the temporal dynamics of the fluid distribution, for this influences the anesthetic effect, the duration of the effect, and, most of all, the additional effects of the TLA solution on the tissue being treated. Only if all these aspects are properly taken into account are the proven great safety and low complication rate assured.

The tumescence caused by the infiltration of the solution is influenced by various factors arising from the volume of TLA, the infiltration time, and the anesthesia waiting time after infiltration as well as individual patient-specific physical conditions. To achieve optimal tumescence these factors must be taken into account. Merely injecting a bag of TLA solution does not mean that one has brought about a genuine, effective tumescence, something that is closely dependent on technique and on making allowance for the particular characteristics of each patient.

As mentioned above in Sect. 9.1, the infiltration rate is variable and partly depends on what is comfortable for the patient. The main factor affecting how uncomfortable a rapid rise in pressure feels is the natural, inherent firmness of the tissue itself.

The tissue changes after infiltration of TLA occurs in three phases:
1. In the first couple of minutes, the injected fluid brings about hydrodissection of the tissue.
2. This is followed by the phase of septal, paralobar fluid distribution in the fatty tissue (up to 20 min).
3. With even longer delay (1/2–1 h), TLA solution starts to diffuse into clusters of cells; in the fatty tissue there is intralobular fluid distribution.

The infiltration rate, the related increase in pressure, and the waiting time all influence the distribution of TLA in the tissue. For this reason, different diffusion rates are advisable for different indications. For example, for skin flaps it makes sense to exploit the hydrodissective effect of the early phase (starting surgery shortly after infiltration), whereas for liposuction, anesthesia waiting times of 1/2–1 h may be appropriate, in order to profit fully from the "lipolytic" effect.

Recommendations and handy hints on injection technique and anesthesia waiting time are given in the respective chapters in Part C.

10 Technique of Subcutaneous Infusion Anesthesia

H. BREUNINGER

10.1 Introduction

When using TLA, for many procedures it is better to infuse the anesthetic solution more slowly than usual, since this means that the patient feels neither pain or pressure. Slow infusion, because it takes longer, also leads to improved surface anesthesia. By using a volumetric infusion pump instead of a roll pump, it is for the first time possible to use this slow, painless, subcutaneous distribution of infusion solution, like a paravenous infusion, for local anesthesia in all operations without having to have a doctor guide the needle all the time (Fig. 10.1). This broadens the range of indications for local anesthesia, especially for children (Fig. 10.2) and for procedures in sensitive parts of the body (Fig. 10.10).

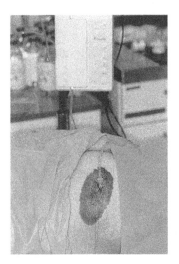

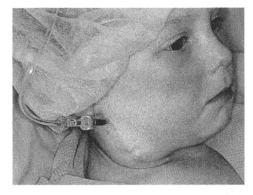

Fig. 10.2. Status after subcutaneous automatic infusion in the neck of a 3-year-old girl with a sebaceous nevus (27-gauge needle, flow 280 ml/h).

Fig. 10.1. Automatic subcutaneous infusion from a central position (injected just subdermally) for partial excision of a congenital nevus (24-gauge needle, flow 400 ml/h). The anesthetic fluid slowly diffuses subcutaneously in all directions

10.2 Method

10.2.1 Pump Requirements

Ordinary volumetric infusion pumps with adjustable flow rate and volume restriction are required (Fresenius INKA ST, flow 0–1500 ml/h, Fig. 10.1, or IVAC 591, flow 0–1000 ml/h). An extension piece is attached to the supplier's infusion set (Fig. 10.3). Several machines can be used on one patient at the same time (Figs. 10.4, 10.10).

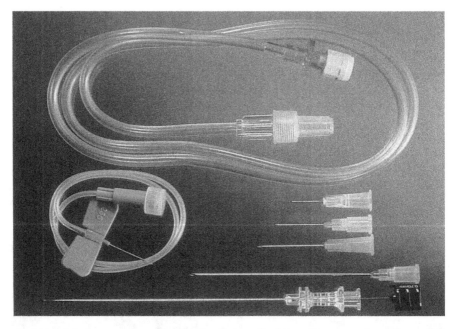

Fig. 10.3. Infusion extension piece and the used needles (30- to 22-gauge or butterfly needles of 27- to 21-gauge, and two spinal needles)

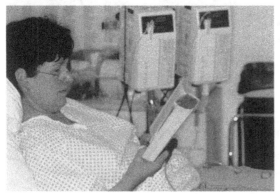

Fig. 10.4. Two or more volumetric infusion pumps can be used if several areas are to be anesthetized. If the procedure is lengthy, the patient can occupy him-/herself with a book

10.2.2 Cannulas

Ordinary cannulas of 30–22 gauge or butterfly needles of 27–21 gauge with a length of 10–100 mm are used (Fig. 10.3). From one to three punctures usually suffice. The injection is done with the infusion solution already flowing. In stripping operations, four to six punctures along the veins are necessary. In these cases, a short manual subcutaneous infusion anesthesia (SIA) using a 30-gauge needle (about 180 ml/h) is carried out first at the site where the spinal needle is to be placed. Small stab incisions are made in the area of the axilla and the groin, into which the [Sprotte] peridural needle is inserted

10.2.3 Anesthetic Solution

See Chap. 3.

10.2.4 Infusion Depth

In normal skin surface surgery, the needle is placed directly under the dermis (Figs. 10.5, 10.6). For a planned high saphenous ligation or groin or axillary dissection, an additional deep infiltration is necessary (Fig. 10.7 and 1) (see Sect. 12.16).

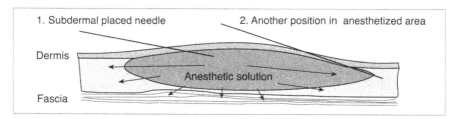

Fig. 10.5. Infusion technique

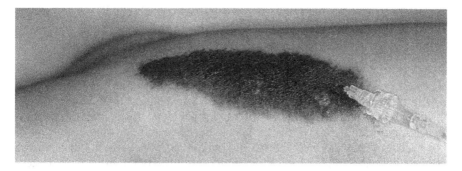

Fig. 10.6. Example of a slow automatic subcutaneous infusion of the anesthetic starting in the first proximal third of the skin alteration (effect of infusion anesthesia); later on, one or two further injections are placed distally in the anesthetized area along the nevus

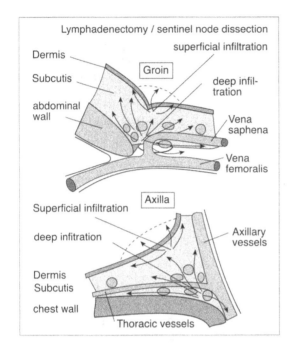

Fig. 10.7. Technique of deep infusion in the axilla and groin

10.2.5 Infusion Volumes

The volumes range from 1 to 1000 ml, depending on the concentration of the solution (see Chap. 3). The volumes needed are always larger than in conventional local anesthesia. Automatic volume restriction (10–250 ml) by the infusion pump is an advantage in order to avoid overinfusion. From time to time, the needle can be moved within the infused area in order to reach areas that still need to be infused without causing further injection pain (Fig. 13.4, Chap. 13). For high saphenous ligation and groin and axillary dissection, first 200 ml are infused superficially in a fan-shaped fashion, then another 200–300 ml into the deeper layers.

10.2.6 Flow Rate

The flow rate varies, depending on the cannula gauge (maximum about 180 ml/h with a 30-gauge cannula, about 350 ml/h with a 27-gauge cannula, about 600 ml/h with a 25-gauge cannula, and about 1500 ml/h with a 22-gauge cannula), the localization, and the extent of the surgery, between 40 and 600 ml/h in the area of the head and neck and between 150 and 1500 ml/h in the body. It is slow during automatic infusion and fast when the cannula is guided by the surgeon. In the case of a obstructionand/or too high pressure an alarm goes off, the flow rate must be reduced and/or the position of the needle point must be altered.

10.2.7 Waiting Period

Depending on the flow rate and the concentration of the anesthetic, one should wait for at least 3 min after ending the infusion at high concentrations and up to a maximum of 0.5–1 h at low concentrations. Very dilute solutions and a short waiting period require additional anesthesia at the injection site, which is not experienced as being painful after the prior infusion.

10.2.8 Medication

A preoperative oral administration of 1 mg flunitrazepam (Rohypnol) has proven to be effective. Perioperative treatment with diazepam analogues given orally or intravenously is only given to anxious patients, or routinely to those undergoing groin or axillary dissection. Prophylactic antibiotic treatment is not given except in cases of already infected wounds. Patients undergoing vein surgery are also given low-molecular-weight heparin.

10.2.9 Monitoring

Pulse oximetry monitoring is necessary. In a slow SIA, the doctor can set up the system and and then leave the patient after about 2 min. With automatic infusion of the groin and axillary, supervision by the OR staff is necessary (Fig. 13.1, Chap. 13) and is appropriate with superficial infusions.

10.3 Further Comments

On the one hand, SIA replaces ordinary local anesthesia, since, even in small operations, no human hand can inject as evenly and slowly as a volumetric infusion pump (Fig. 10.8). On the other hand, it is equivalent to tumescent anesthesia when large areas are infiltrated (Fig. 10.9). This injection technique allows local anesthesia without pain, making it possible to employ local anesthesia even in very

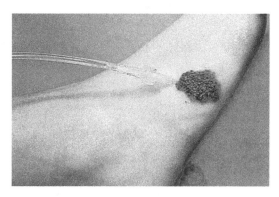

Fig. 10.8. Even for small skin alterations, SIA is less painful for the patient and less time-consuming for the doctor, since it is infused automatically

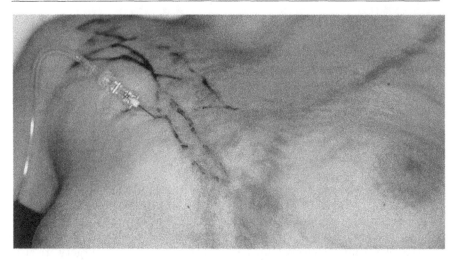

Fig. 10.9. Use of SIA in an extended scar correction. The fluid is also distributed beneath scars, although the anesthetic effect must be closely checked before surgery begins

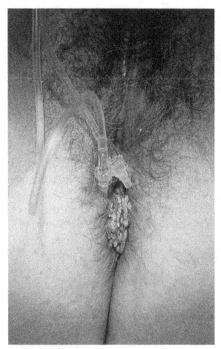

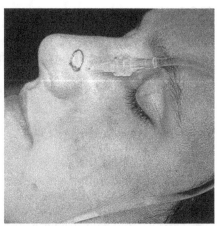

Fig. 10.11. In the sensitive nasal area the anesthetic solution is distributed continuously: in this case infusion with a 30-gauge needle at a flow rate of 60 ml/h

Fig. 10.10. In very sensitive areas, too, the use of SIA is a relief for the patient: in this case slow infusion (150 ml/h) using a 30-gauge needle for treatment of condylomata accuminata

sensitive parts of the body (Fig. 10.10) and for operations more usually carried out under general anesthesia (see Fig. 13.1). Generally, one can say: The smaller the planned operation, the higher the concentration, the thinner the cannula, and the slower the flow rate (especially in the area of the nose, Fig. 10.11) and vice versa. Underinfusion should be avoided at all costs.

SIA can be done manually or run automatically via an infusion pump. In the latter case, the doctor can turn his/her attention to other things for the duration of the infusion. Slow infusion without the doctor present often has a very calming effect, especially on children and sensitive patients (see Figs. 13.1–4). During the infusion, the patient can lie in bed and read (Fig. 10.4), listen to music, or watch a video. It is advantageous to have a special room for this, and we have equipped our recovery room accordingly.

Even in small operations, the patients report feeling significantly less pain than with conventional injections. Advance planning and timely induction of the SIA are very important for the smooth running of the operation, but this is not normally a problem so long as a pre-op room is available.

SIA using prilocaine diluted by Ringer's solution, is an economic, safe, and extremely low-pain method of anesthesia for almost all kinds of surgery on the skin, especially in children and sensitive patients. It does, however, require a certain amount of experience.

References

1. Acosta AE (1997) Clinical parameters of tumescent anesthesia in skin cancer reconstructive surgery. A review of 86 patients. Arch Dermatol 133:451–454
2. Auletta MJ (1993) New developements in local anesthesia. In: Roenigk RK, Roenigk HH (eds) Surgical dermatology. Mosby-Year Book, St Louis pp 7–8
3. Coleman WP, Klein JA (1992) Use of the tumescent technique for scalp surgery, dermabrasion and soft tissue reconstruction. J Dermatol Surg Oncol 18:130–135
4. Goodman G (1994) Dermabrasion using tumescent anesthesia. J Dermatol Surg Oncol 20:802–807
5. Hanke CW, Bernstein G, Bullock S (1996) Safety of tumescent liposuction in 15,336 patients-national survey results. J Dermatol Surg Oncol 21:459–462
6. Ilouz RG (1983) Body contouring by lipolysis: a 5 year experience with over 3000 cases. Plast Reconst Surg 72:591–595
7. Janer GL, Padial M, Sanchez IL (1993) Less painful alternatives for local anesthesia. J Dermatol Surg Oncol 19:237–240
8. Klein JA (1987) The tumescent technique for liposuction surgery. Am J Cosm Surg 4:263–267
9. Klein JA (1990) Tumescent technique for regional anesthesia permits lidocaine doses of 35 mg/kg for liposuction. J Dermatol Surg Oncol 16:248–263
10. Lillis PJ (1990) The tumescent technique for liposuction surgery. In: Lillis PJ, Coleman WP (eds) Dermatologic clinics. Saunders, Philadelphia, 439–50
11. Mc Kay N, Morris R, Mushlin P (1987) Sodium bicarbonate attenuates pain on skin infiltration with lidocaine, with or without epinephrine. Anesth Analg 66:572–576
12. Ostad A, Kageyama N, Moy RL (1996) Tumescent anesthesia with lidocaine dose of 55 mg/kg is safe for liposuction. J Dermatol Surg Oncol 22:921–927
13. Smith SL, Hodge JA, Lawrence N, et al. (1992) The importance of bicarbonate in large volume anesthetic preparations. J Dermatol Surg Oncol 18:973–975
14. Thompson KD, Welykyj S, Massa MC (1993) Antibacterial activity of lidocaine in combination with a bicarbonate buffer. J Dermatol Surg Oncol 19:216–220

11 Patient Selection and Preoperative Preparation

D. BERGFELD, B. SOMMER

As already demonstrated, TLA is a very safe method. Because of its various advantages, it is often suitable for patients in whom intubation anesthesia and other forms of anesthesia are contraindicated (see Chap. 4). Nonetheless, with TLA as with other methods, patients must be carefully selected with regard to physical and psychological characteristics and their suitability for the treatment, if the method is to be used as safely as possible.

11.1 Are There Contraindications for TLA?

The only absolute contraindication is a known allergy to the anesthetic in the solution. When 50-ml bottles are used, a para group allergy must also be considered, since these package sizes contain parahydroxybenzonic acid as a preservative.

Special caution and appropriate supervision are necessary in patients with marked myocardial weakness because of the danger of volume overload from the resorbed fluid, and also in patients with a known tendency to high-grade cardiac arrhythmia or paroxysmal tachycardia, because of the proarrhythmic effect of the local anesthetic. Patients with these preexisting conditions must be monitored very closely (pulse, blood pressure, signs of overhydration, ECG monitoring).

In patients with liver function disorders, the clearance of lidocaine may be severely impaired, since this local anesthetic is mostly metabolized by the liver. Prilocaine is excreted via the lung in addition, which makes it safer.

Because it leads to methemoglobin formation, prilocaine should not be used in the following risk groups: premature babies and neonates, and patients with a glucose-6-phosphate-dehydrogenase deficiency (anamnesis). As a general principle, extra caution is required in patients from Southern Europe because of the possibility of an existing glucose-6-phosphate-dehydrogenase defect [3]. Another contraindication to using prilocaine is concurrent administration of other substances that form methemoglobin. Examples of such substances are chlorates and the nitrites and sulfonamides used in coronary heart disease.

Psychologically unstable patients and those with an extreme fear of needles and injections are basically unsuited to TLA. In these cases, the decision on whether to use it or not should be made jointly with the patient on a case-by-case basis, after comprehensive discussion and explanation of the technique.

11.2 What Preliminary Tests Are Necessary?

The preliminary tests required vary, depending on the extent of the planned procedure.

A detailed history must be obtained for each patient in regard to preexisting conditions of the CNS, heart, lung, liver, kidneys, and thyroid function disorders. The following have significance for extended TLA [2]:

- CNS – Tendency to seizures, since high concentrations of local anesthetic can provoke seizures.
- Heart – In cases of serious heart disease, such as coronary heart disease, a history of myocardial infarction, cardiac insufficiency, and the like, an internist should be consulted.
- Lung – Important factors are a tendency to bronchospasm and excessive smoking.
- Gastrointestinal tract – Stomach ulcers may enlarge in response to the stress of surgery. Liver damage inhibits metabolism of the local anesthetic.
- Kidney – Renal insufficiency can lead to retention of fluid and metabolites.
- Muscles, bones, and joints – In patients with spinal syndromes, back pain may be exacerbated by long sessions on the OR table.

The patient should be asked about current medication as well as existing allergies or infectious diseases (hepatitis, HIV).

The physical exam is necessary in order to get an overview of the patient's health condition and to check on the important organ functions. If sedation is considered, blood pressure and the results of heart and lung auscultation should be documented. Especially for cosmetic procedures, dermatologic evaluation of the skin complexion, scars, and pigmented spots is mandatory.

In all procedures with TLA, current laboratory results regarding electrolytes (because of the increased risk of cardiac arrhythmias with electrolyte disorders), liver and kidney values, and coagulation status should be at hand [2].

It has been shown that routine ECG and chest x-rays do not increase perioperative safety. Only in cases where the history and detailed physical exam indicate a possible increased perioperative risk, does a differentiated preoperative test program become necessary [4].

One aid to risk evaluation is the classification produced by the American Society of Anesthesiology (ASA):

1. Normal, healthy patient
2. Patient with slight generalized debility but without restriction of performance, e.g. slight bronchial asthma
3. Patient with severe generalized debility with restriction of performance
4. Patient inactivated by general debility which poses a threat to life
5. Moribund patient

Cosmetic procedures should only be performed in patients in categories 1 and 2.

11.3   What Safety Precautions Should Be Available?

The treatment of reactions to local anesthetics may require the clearing of airways, administration of oxygen or ventilation, placement of an infusion, or restoring circulation by external cardiac massage.

It is a principle that large amounts of local anesthetic should not be given without the presence of an indwelling venous catheter, a stand-by source of oxygen, suction device, mask, ventilation bag, laryngoscope, and tracheal tubes as well as any medication that might be needed (sedatives, vagolytics, corticosteroids, antihistamines, epinephrine).

In extended procedures in patients with a relevant history, even local anesthesia requires monitoring by ECG and pulse oximetry.

References

1. Diem E (1993) Anästhesiologische Voraussetzungen ambulanten und tageschirurgischen Operierens. In: Winter H, Bellmann K-P (eds) Fortschritte der operativen und onkologischen Dermatologie, vol 9. Springer, Berlin Heidelberg New York pp 91–96
2. Klein JA (1997) Anesthesia for dermatologic surgery. In: Coleman WP, Hanke CW, Alt TH, Asken S, Mosby (eds) Cosmetic surgery of the skin. Mosby, St Louis, pp 62–70
3. Reinhard M (1993) Regionalanästhesieverfahren. In: Reinhard M, Schaefer R (eds) Klinikleitfaden Anästhesie. Jungjohann, Neckarsulm, pp 292–299
4. Thoens M, Zenz M (1997) Vorbereitung des Patienten zur Regionalanästhesie. Anästhesiologie und Intensivmedizin. 9:464–469

Part C

Indications

12 Liposuction

B. SOMMER, G. SATTLER

As already demonstrated in previous chapters, liposuction has played a leading role in the history of the development of TLA, since the method was initially developed especially for this indication, and much knowledge and further development have been based on experiences and studies in liposuction.

Definition

Liposuction is the surgical suction of circumscribed fat accumulations by selective removal of adipocytes with the aid of sturdy cannulas. The current suction cannulas have an outer diameter of 1.5–4 mm and have a variable number of holes on the front, normally blunt, end.

History

The method of suction of subcutaneous fat with suction needles was developed by Georgio and Arpad Fischer in Rome in the mid 1970s. They had a machine which enabled them to suction out unprepared fat with hollow needles under general anesthesia [10]. This procedure was not without risk because of the severe blood loss and the anesthetic risks, and the cosmetic result was often unsatisfactory because of irregularities and dents (see Chap. 2).

The next important advances which aided further spreading of the method came from Gerard Illouz in Paris. In addition to using new suction devices, he introduced the so called "wet technique." This involved injecting saline solution mixed with hyaluronidase into the fat. It became apparent that this reduced blood loss and facilitated the suction [15].

On the basis of this "wet technique" and under professional/political pressure aimed at restricting the activities of surgical dermatologists to outpatient procedures that can be performed under local anesthetic, the pharmacologist and dermatologist Jeffrey Klein developed TLA in California in the late 1980s. By adding lidocaine, epinephrine, and sodium bicarbonate to physiologic saline solution, he achieved sufficient local anesthesia when injecting into the suction areas.

In 1987, he published his first experiences with the tumescent solution he had developed [16] (Table 12.1).

The technique of TLA revolutionized liposuction [5]. Even in those early days, the great advantages of this method were obvious: no need for risky general

Component	Amount
Lidocaine 1%	50.0 ml
Epinephrine 1:10,000	1.0 ml
Sodium bicarbonate 8.4%	12.5 ml
Triamcinolone–acetonide	10 mg
NaCl 0.9%	1000 ml

Table 12.1. Klein's tumescent solution

anesthesia, significantly reduced blood loss, immediate patient mobilization, and significantly shorter convalescence.

In the course of time, various research groups modified the composition and recommended volumes of the solution developed by Klein (see Sect. 3.6). In Europe, lidocaine was replaced by prilocaine, which causes less systemic toxicity [27], although it does cause formation of methemoglobin (see Chap. 5).

At the same time, to reach the high safety attainable by this method, it is necessary to stick to the recommended doses, techniques, and time factors (anesthesia "waiting time"), as well as appropriate follow-up and possible concomitant medications for infection and thrombosis prevention (see Chap. 7).

The proven safe use of higher total volumes of local anesthetic given at lower concentrations in the TLA solution made it possible to use significantly larger amounts of TLA and thus to treat ever larger and more extensive areas in one session. Whereas early on only up to 2 l Klein tumescent solution was used, which is only sufficient for the treatment of very limited areas (e.g., only riding breeches deformity or only medial thigh), 6–8 l TLA solution can be safely infiltrated today. This makes it possible to treat several areas in one session.

However, to guarantee the effect and the safety of TLA, one should always be careful to bring the areas to be suctioned up to a sufficiently tumescent state without at the same time exceeding the recommended upper limits of TLA volume.

Concept of Physiodynamic Tumescence

The experience gained in the course of tumescent liposuction over the years has led to the development of a model of the processes that take place in the fat after TLA which may explain the good results of this method.

The goal of liposuction is suction of pure adipose tissue. Connective tissue, lymph and blood vessels, and skin nerves should be spared as much as possible. The destruction of blood vessels may lead to severe blood loss and hematoma formation. Extensive damage to lymph vessels can result in edema and seromas. The connective tissue of the fatty tissue constitutes a stabilizing framework that needs to be preservedand plays an important role in the postoperative wound contraction. If it is destroyed during surgery, the skin can no longer be pulled tight to the underlying layers and remains flaccid.

The TLA solution first causes hydrodissection of the tissue. The next step is a paraseptal or paralobular distribution pattern, followed finally by intralobular diffusion (see Chap. 9). This means that, if one waits long enough, the fat becomes softened, the fat cell lobules become separated from each other to a certain extent, and this allows the adipocytes to be suctioned off gently and evenly. The result is markedly reduced trauma to the blood vessels and connective tissue. In addition, the high tissue pressure that is obtained after tumescence has been reached further reduces the shearing forces caused by the movements of the suction cannula.

The above-mentioned tissue changes caused by TLA have made it possible in the last few years to use ever finer suction cannulas. Starting in 1994, cannulas were used for suctioning which until then had only been used to infiltrate the tumescent solution.

At the beginning of 1997, in collaboration with Dr. G. Blugerman, we introduced a blunt suction cannula (diameter 2–4 mm) with 24 suction holes arranged circularly. This was based on the observation that too much connective tissue was always removed with the conventional needles; as could be seen on endoscopic imaging as well as during lipotransfer or liporecycling. The rationale of this development was as follows: if the suction of about 0.9 Pa produced by the mechanical suction device is applied to only one opening, then all of the suction takes place there. Distribution of the suction force among many holes reduces the force effective at each hole. Thus, in a 24-hole cannula, only 1/24 of the applied suction force will be effective at each hole, i.e., a little under 0.04 bar (see Fig. 12.1). This is just enough to loosen the fat calls in a well established tumescence, but too weak to destroy larger connective tissue fibers.

The circular arrangement of the holes, which measure 0.9 and 1.2 mm in diameter, enables self-regulated distribution of the suction pressure, for if the holes on one side are obstructed by connective tissue structures or, by the dermis, no violent force can be applied to the tissue, since the holes on the other side are suctioning soft pliable adipose tissue.

As an analogy, imagine a water hose on which, out of a total of 24 holes, 6 on one side are to be held shut. This will be quite easy to do, unlike trying to hold shut 2 out of 2 holes positioned on the same side, because in this case the fall water pressure will be pushing against both of the holes. Going back to the suction cannula, this explains the relatively low trauma caused by the same suction force. This enables even more accurate work, and will thus give improved cosmetic results.

Doing Without General Anesthesia

With TLA extensive areas can be sufficiently anesthetized without the need for other methods of anesthesia [19, 28]. This is described in Chap. 4.

Great Intraoperative Safety

The great safety of TLA in liposuctions has been proven in a study with a very large number of patients. In 1995, Hanke et al. published the results of a patient survey in the US relating to liposuction performed under TLA (for a list of complications, see Table 12.2). Data collected on more than 15,000 patients showed not a single instance of a severe complication (death, lung embolism, massive blood loss with hypovolemic shock). None of the patients needed a blood transfusion. Tumescent liposuction can therefore be regarded as an extremely safe method [13, 14].

Complications

The following rather common but not severe complications have been reported and should be mentioned to the patient in the information session before a planned liposuction (see Table 12.2): transient edematous swelling, e.g., of the scrotum or the labia due to the TLA solution (0.3847%), very rarely persisting edema (0.0978%), infections (0.3391%), persisting skin unevenness, dents (0.2608%), hematomas and seromas (0.1695%), circumscribed panniculitis-like skin reactions and thickening (0.1956%), allergic reactions to medications or dressings (0.1174%), and vasovagal reactions/syncopes (0.0717%).

Thrombophlebitis did not occur in the patients studied by Hanke et al., but has been occasionally observed by us. In the area of the medial thigh and the medial side of the knee, especially, an insufficient long saphenous vein may be affected detrimentally. Healthy blood vessels normally tolerate the trauma caused by the suction without problems, especially when they are to a large extent protected from shearing forces by firm tumescence. Venous insufficiency must be checked for in the obligatory physical exam during the patient information session, and if there is any ground for suspicion, a complete phlebologic examination should be carried out.

The risk of a *deep vein thrombosis* in the leg is not specifically discussed in the Hanke study; no case of lung embolism occurred. We have only observed deep vein thrombosis of the leg in patients with a family history of frequent thromboses. The thrombosis risk as such is in many ways minimized by the tumescent technique:

- Vascular and muscle tone are unchanged during the procedure, in contrast to the case with the relaxants used in general anesthesia.
- Patient mobilization starts already during the operation, since the patient usually goes to the bathroom between the TLA infiltration and the beginning of surgery, often has to change position during the surgery ("multipositional liposuction"), and in addition stands up near the end of the operation so that the symmetry of the result can be assessed.
- The tumescent solution has an antithrombotic effect in itself, since probably any local anesthetic of the amide type has antithrombotic properties [29].
  - The strongly hemostatic effect of the tumescent solution greatly reduces the risk of *bleeding*. Because of the immense blood loss that occurred in early liposuctions – at a 1:1 ratio to the suctioned fat – autologous blood transfusions were almost always necessary [7,11]. With correctly performed tumescent liposuction technique, the blood loss is about 1% of the total aspirate [17,18,20].

Medical Indications for Liposuction

Launois–Bensaude benign symmetric lipomatosis

Benign symmetric lipomatosis is a rare disease of adipose tissue, the etiology of which is unknown; pathogenetically it is probably caused by a localized defect of catecholamine-induced lipolysis. It is often associated with alcoholism, hepatopathy, glucose intolerance, hyperuricemia, and malignant tumors of the upper airways, which is why a thorough clinical exam is mandatory.

Table 12.2. Complications in 15,336 patients who underwent liposuction under TLA (adapted from [16])

Complication	Number of patients	%
Scrotal or labial edema	59	0.3847
Infection	52	0.3391
Persistent irregularities in the skin relief	40	0.2608
Postoperative focal subcutaneous panniculitis-like reactions	30	0.1956
Hematoma/seromas	26	0.1695
Allergic reaction to accompanying medication or adhesive tape	18	0.1174
Persistent postoperative edema	15	0.0978
Patient dissatisfaction due to unrealistic expectations	13	0.0848
Nausea not associated with other analgesics	11	0.0717
Vasovagal reaction or syncope	11	0.0717
Permanent hyper- or hypopigmentation	6	0.0391
Excessive or persistent postoperative pain	9	0.0587
Postoperative fever	8	0.0522
Abnormally extended ecchymoses	5	0.0326
Unusual postoperative sleepiness/tiredness	5	0.0326
Permanent damage to sensitive nerves	5	0.0326
Cardiac arrhythmias requiring treatment	2	0.0130
Anemia	0	0
Complications requiring hospitalization	0	0
Blood or fluid losses requiring transfusions	0	0
Venous embolism or fat embolism	0	0
Hypovolemic shock	0	0
Perforation of peritoneum or thorax	0	0
Seizures	0	0
Thrombophlebitis	0	0
Toxic reactions to intravenous sedative or narcotic	0	0
Death	0	0

Today, cosmetic and functional improvement of benign symmetric lipomatosis is possible using the technique of liposuction under TLA. Because of the higher proportion of connective tissue structures and blood vessels, the procedure is more difficult and the amount of fat extracted is less than in the suction of circumscribed fat accumulations in cosmetic liposuction. For these reasons, the aspirate contains significantly more blood [26].

Madelung's Disease

Madelung's disease is the cervical form of benign symmetric lipomatosis [23]. While some authors still prefer invasive surgical treatment, even after the introduction of liposuction [1, 21], the latter performed under well-established TLA has proven its worth in our experience and that of other authors [8]. Here, too, relatively little fat (compared to the case in normal lipohypertrophy) can be suctioned in each session. If this is taken into account when planning the surgery, however, significant success can be achieved in the course of a few sessions (Figs. 12.3–12.6).

Buffalo Hump in Cushing's Syndrome

The "buffalo hump" fat accumulations so burdensome to the patient with Cushing's syndrome can be very satisfactorily treated with liposuction under TLA. Here, the fat is softer than in benign symmetric lipomatosis, and the postoperative retraction of the skin causes no problems.

Lipomatosis dolorosa (Dercum's Disease)

Dercum's disease is also treated with intravenous lidocaine, so an obvious step is to inject lidocaine in the Klein solution directly into the painful subcutaneous tissue and then in addition reduce the mass of the tissue by liposuction. However, no very striking success has materialized so far among our patients with Dercum's disease; the pain was slightly relieved. Observations in larger series have yet to be made.

Hypertrophic Insulin Lipodystrophy

As in all other lipohypertrophies, the adipose tissue in hypertrophic insulin lipodystrophy is easily accessible to liposuction and can be satisfactorily removed.

Partial Lipodystrophy Syndrome

The special feature of this disease is that areas of lipohypertrophy exist next to lipoatrophy, causing marked bumpiness and unevenness in the skin which is naturally very upsetting for the affected person. In these cases, a combination of liposuction in the hypertrophic or pseudohypertrophic areas and fat injection into atrophic areas is a solution. The fat harvested in the liposuction is recycled under sterile conditions and reinjected into the subcutis as for an autologous fat transfer. There are several techniques for liporecycling; a description of a method in connection with tumescent liposuction can be found in Sattler and Sommer [25].

Hemifacial Atrophy (Romberg's Disease)

In this disease, great success can be achieved using the technique of fat transfer. The technique for reinjection of fat does not differ from that in other fat transplantations. The "life span" of the transplanted fat cannot be exactly predicted, however, since a variable percentage of it is absorbed and metabolized by the body [3, 12]. Because of the rich blood supply to the facial area, there is a danger, although slight, of ocular and cerebral fat embolism. This complication has never been observed by us, but has been reported in the literature [9]. For this reason, fat reinjections in the face should be carried out especially slowly. In general, all fat transplantations carry the risk of (pseudo-) cyst formation, which increases with the amount of tissue deposited at one site. Therefore, it is always advisable to use micro fat injection, which means the injection of very small fat droplets.

Fat Transplantation to Treat Sunken Excision Sites Covered with Split-Thickness Grafts After Removal of Malignant Melanoma

With the technique of liporecycling (fat transfer) mentioned above, even large, deep defects, e.g. after excision of melanomas followed by split-thickness skin grafts after insufficient granulation, can be corrected. Because a varying percentage of the transplanted fat is resorbed, several sessions may sometimes be necessary.

Lipolymphedema

If liposuction is performed correctly under TLA only [22], the lymph vessels are to a large extent spared. Therefore, it is also possible to treat combinations of fat hypertrophy and diseases of the lymph vessels today. The ratio of injected TLA solution and suctioned adipose tissue should always be lower than 1:1 in order to achieve sufficient stretching of the subcutaneous space and to minimize the shear forces.

Pseudogynecomastia and Gynecomastia

The male breast contains more fibrous tissue than other body areas. Therefore, suction of gynecomastia is only possible with very small cannulas; the results are sometimes very good, though [4].

Breast Reduction

On the use of liposuction in breast reduction, see Sect. 25.

Fat Removal from Transposition Flaps and Correction of Skin Flaps

Insufficiently defatted transposition and rotation flaps may be defatted later with the aid of liposuction, if they are large enough. This spares the patient and the surgeon further open surgery [6, 27].

Cosmetic Indications for Liposuction

As already mentioned, liposuction was developed to remove cosmetically undesirable circumscribed fat deposits. All subcutaneous fat accumulations are suitable for this treatment, but deeper, intra-abdominal, fat depots are not accessible. Depending on the gynecoid or android fat distribution type [30], social orientation, current ideals of beauty, accumulations of adipose tissue, either genetically determined or resulting from hyperalimentation, are felt to be disturbing, and surgical aid is sought for their removal.

Liposuction is the most common cosmetic surgical procedure in the USA. According to statistics from the American Academy of Cosmetic Surgery (AACS, Executive Office, 401 N. Michigan Avenue, Chicago, IL 60611, USA) a total of 292,942 liposuctions were performed in the US in 1996, of which 238,836 were in women and 54,106 in men, and the trend is rising.

According to the same statistics, the three most often corrected body regions are, in order of frequency:
- In women: abdomen, thigh, and flank
- In men: abdomen, flanks, and "love handles" (midriff rolls)

Body regions can also be classified according to their suitability to undergo liposuction, since the healing process and retractability of the skin vary not only interindividually, but intraindividually depending on the body region.
- Body regions well suited to liposuction are: neck, male breast, waist, abdomen, medial side of the knee, ankle, and calf.
- Above-average skin retraction can be expected in the following regions: cheeks, upper arms, hips, riding breeches, lateral and suprapatellar sides of the knee.
- Average skin retraction can be expected in the following regions: back, upper abdomen, pubic region, medial and proximal thigh, and outer aspects of the buttocks.
- Generally poor skin retraction is seen in the following regions: front of the thighs, axilla, and inner aspects of the buttocks.

In general, a diffuse lobular fibrosis develops after suctioning, due to the more or less even damage to the subcutaneous fat. This fibrosis is different from fibrosis of other etiologies [2]. The diffuse fibrosis connected to the wound healing process is the primary cause for the skin reaction.

Patient Information

Every planned liposuction under TLA should be preceded by a detailed patient information session. A patient who has understood the specific advantages of the method will cooperate better. The risks outlined above should be represented in a manner appropriate to their frequency.

The patient should also be made aware of the following:
- Increasing swelling and hematoma formation is normal in the first few days after surgery.
- Fluid drainage of the TLA solution continues for 2–3 days after the procedure. Here also, a well-informed patient will better tolerate this quite positive side effect (wash-out of hematomas, decreased risk of infection).
- Increasing firmness and swelling in the abdominal area (may persist for up to 3 months).
- Further corrections may be necessary (3–5 % of cases).

12.1 Technique

The intended treatment objective and the extent of the planned procedure are decided during the preoperative interview. The amount of TLA solution required is the factor that determines the extent of each operative session and whether several sessions will be needed in order to reach the desired treatment result.

A photo documentation should always be made prior to the surgery itself. After this, the surgical site is marked with a colored pen. Depending on need, additional oral, intravenous, or intramuscular medication can be given (see Chap. 6).

We routinely insert an intravenous catheter. The more additional medications that are given, especially centrally acting substances, the more necessary continuous monitoring by pulse oximetry, regular blood pressure checks, and maybe even ECG monitoring appears [14]. In our experience, these measures are usually unnecessary if the use of additional medications is restrained and the guidelines regarding amounts of TLA solution are strictly observed.

After skin disinfection, subcutaneous wheals containing 1% local anesthetic (about 5–10 ml) are distributed such that tumescence can be induced painlessly throughout the whole surgical site by fan-shaped infiltration from these sites.

As shown in Chap. 9, various possible infiltration techniques exist. Since the area to be made tumescent is usually quite large, a mechanical infiltration technique is recommended, i.e., infiltration aided by a pump system. If an infiltration cannula is used, the infiltration rate can be varied according to the area and the patient's subjective perception (the tighter the tissue, the more uncomfortable a rapid increase in pressure is felt to be) [22]. We have had very good experiences with the Sattler distributor, which distributes the TLA solution via several cannulas at different sites at the same time (see Figs. 9.9 and 12.2). With this technique, pressure builds up slowly at each cannula, while at the same time excellent tumescence is quickly achieved. On the other hand, working with several cannulas at once does require some familiarization on the part of the treating person.

During the infiltration, one must make sure that enough TLA is distributed into the deeper layers early on. If one stays too close to the surface in the beginning, it becomes virtually impossible to reach the deeper layers through the tumescent superficial areas.

As in all tumescent infiltration procedures, the tissue turgor must be constantly monitored by palpation.

TLA Technique in Benign Fat Diseases

This technique does not differ much from that in liposuction for cosmetic indications.

Surgical planning must include the decision on which areas can be treated in one session, which in turn depends on the assessment, based on experience, of how much tumescent solution will be needed.

The preoperative preparations are like those for liposuctions. Especially where findings are very asymmetric, precise preoperative markings are important.

Depending on the underlying disease, the degree of fibrosis and the composition of the fat can vary considerably, which may influence the course of the infiltration and suction. Slightly fibrotic tissue is easier to infiltrate and suction, so the waiting time for the tumescent solution can be shorter. A higher proportion of connective tissue, manifest as increased resistance, makes the infiltration lengthy, and the subsequent suction requires increased caution.

Helpful Hints for the Infiltration of the TLA Solution

- Check the TLA solution carefully before starting the infiltration. Is it ready to be used ? Which nurse mixed it ?
- Check the temperature of the solution. It should be at room temperature at least, warmer if possible.
- Begin the infiltration as slowly as possible and in a less painful area.
- Monitor tissue turgor constantly, visually and by palpation.
- Infiltrate deeper layers first, then superficial ones.
- Adjust the infiltration rate to the anatomic region and the individual patient's pain sensitivity.
- Aim for the fullest tissue turgor possible ("like a watermelon").
- Wait for the blanching effect; determine the waiting time.
- The most common beginner's mistake is to use too little tumescent solution.
- The most common mistake by experienced surgeons is to use too little tumescent solution.

Of course, one has to remember with these given volumes that various individual patient factors contribute significantly to achieving optimal tumescence. In addition to the patient's height, the condition of the tissue being infiltrated also determines the amount of TLA required (see Table 12.3). For example, if 3 l tumescent solution is infiltrated into a 1.80-m-tall patient who has just lost 15 kg in the last few months, this will cause a different tumescent effect, because of the condition the tissue is in, to the effect of the same volume infiltrated into a 1.60-m-tall patient who has just put on 6 kg. Thus, different individual characteristics influence the tumescent effect and should be taken into account in the preoperative planning.

After complete tumescence of the treatment site, which means a bulging hard turgor (watermelon-like), a waiting time from about 20 min to up to an hour is necessary. This allows time for the fat to be optimally softened by the diffusion of TLA solution, and prepared for the suction which will follow (for details of the process see Sect. 12.2 below).

During this anesthesia waiting period, the tumescence loses turgor due to leakage from the injection sites. In order to reduce to a minimum the shearing forces acting on the fat during suction, a little more solution can be reinjected before the liposuction is started. This can be TLA solution if the maximum TLA dose has not been reached yet, otherwise normal saline solution or Ringer's lactate solution may be used.

Table 12.3. Average amount of fluid needed for different body areas	Body part	Amount of fluid
	Abdomen	2000–6000 ml
	Hip	600–2000 ml per side
	Lateral thigh	500–2000 ml per side
	Ventral thigh	600–2000 ml per side
	Medial thigh	600–1500 ml per side
	Medial knee	500– 700 ml per side

Fat prepared in this way can be suctioned very evenly using extremely thin suction cannulas from about 5-mm incisions on the margins of the treated area, sparing the connective tissue and vascular structures. The development of finer cannulas paralleled the development of TLA; currently, we use cannulas with a diameter of 2–4 mm with numerous small openings (see Fig. 12.1).

The cannulas are moved to and fro in the tissue, so that at each movement fat is sucked or "plucked out" through the side holes. It is then drawn through a transparent tube to the suction device. This allows an evaluation of how much blood is being drawn out with it.

The patient, being awake, can be asked to change his/her position during surgery, or to get up so the result of the surgery to be assessed.

After the liposuction has been completed, the incision sites are closed with sterile strips which are covered with a sterile dressing for additional wound protection. Immediately afterwards, a compression dressing is applied, which should be lined with fluid-absorbing cellulose in order to avoid becoming immediately soaked through.

If no centrally acting additional medication has been given, the patient may be discharged from hospital with an escort immediately after surgery if he/she wishes.

Perioperatively, we, like some other surgeons, give prophylactic antibiotic treatment. In patients at risk for thrombosis prophylaxis may also be considered (see Chap. 7).

Follow-up appointments are usually scheduled for 2–3 days later, and signs of infection should be particularly looked for.

12.2 Specific Advantages

The well-known advantages of TLA apply particularly to tumescent liposuction. They have already been mentioned:
- No need for general anesthesia with its attendant risks.
- Great safety owing to reduced blood loss.
- Analgesia lasts longer than the procedure.
- Immediate patient mobilization, significantly more rapid recovery.
- Fewer hematomas.
- An awake patient can change position during the procedure and stand up for the result to be checked.
- Improved cosmetic results.
- Very safe method when carried out correctly.

- Decreased risk of infection because of bacteriostatic effects of local anesthetic and the "washing-out" of the TLA solution through the incisions, inhibiting the ingress of microorganisms.
- Also well suited to ultrasound-guided liposuctions, since heat convection reduces the danger of burns.

12.3   Specific Disadvantages

The outline of the areas to be treated must be well marked, since the landmarks of the body are unrecognizable after infiltration of the tumescent fluid.

Because so much fluid has been introduced, it is more difficult to assess the suctioned region at the end of surgery. The fluid diffuses and runs, especially as drawn by gravity, into the surrounding tissue, and this may cause the suctioned area to sink slightly while the surrounding areas appear swollen. In such a case, one has to rely on palpation to make a judgement.

There is a danger of over-correction because the fat is artificially swollen by the TLA solution. This can suggest a false sense of security on the basis of an increased epidermis–fascia distance; after healing, it may become apparent that inadvertently too much fat has been removed and the transition to the nonsuctioned area is too abrupt.

Disadvantages of TLA in liposuction and possible pitfalls are the following:
Imprecise preoperative marking can lead to assessment errors because the fat is swollen by the TLA solution.

- Risk of oversuctioning, because the bulging tumescent area gives a false sense of security and as a result too much fat is suctioned.
- Risk of hypothermia with arrhythmias or immunosuppression if the TLA solution is too cold.
- Risk of pulmonary edema if additional i.v. fluids are given, since the TLA acts as an interstitial infusion.
- Where findings are extensive, there is a danger of trying to remove too much fat in one session The greater trauma and prolonged surgery time can cancel out some of the advantages and the normally great intraoperative safety of the method.
- Liposuction under TLA cannot be combined with other cosmetic surgical procedures in the same session because risks increase, e.g., the risk of thrombosis becomes much higher.

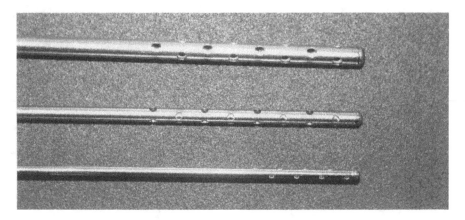

Fig. 12.1. Blugermann-Sattler 24 hole suction cannula. LaserPoint (see part C)

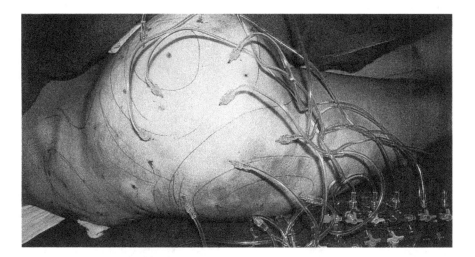

Fig. 12.2. Induction of tumescent local anesthesia with several 20 gg cannulas, in this case using an assemblage of four Sattler distributors. LaserPoint (see part C)

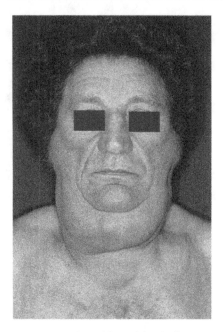

Fig. 12.3. Patient with Madelung's disease, the cervical form of Launois–Bensaude benign symmetric lipomatosis

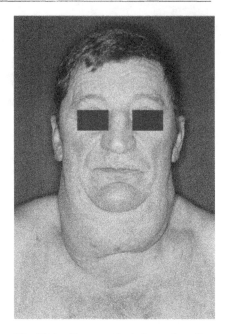

Fig. 12.4. Same patient 6 months after liposuction under TLA

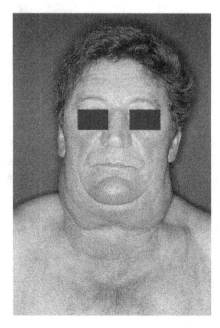

Fig. 12.5. Same patient 6 months after the second liposuction under TLA

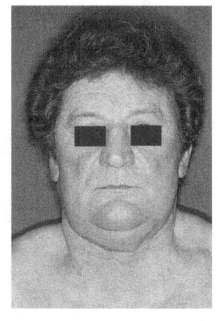

Fig. 12.6. Same patient 6 months after the third liposuction under TLA

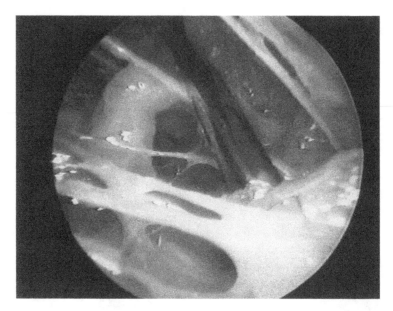

Fig. 12.7. Endoscopic image: normal subcutaneous fat with real connective tissue suspension, the blunt 3-mm diameter suction cannula, and some remaining fat flaps. Especially remarkable is how even quite small strings of connective tissue are preserved

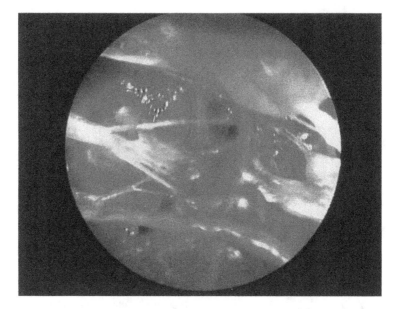

Fig. 12.8. Endoscopic image: normal subcutaneous fat in a patient with Launois–Bensaude benign symmetric lipomatosis, with immense vascularization and increased infiltration by connective tissue

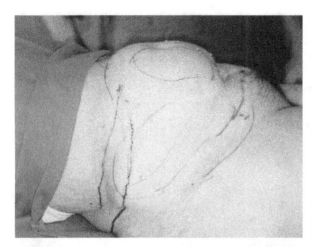

Fig. 12.9. Blanching effect of abdominal tumescence prior to liposuction

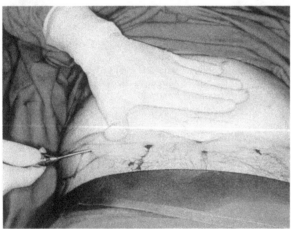

Fig. 12.10. Same patient: suction procedure with stab incision, monitored by palpation with the other hand

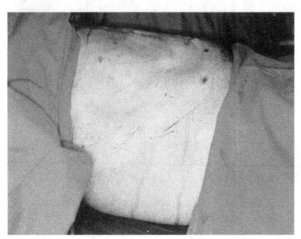

Fig. 12.11. Same patient: immediately postoperative appearance, now with a flat abdominal contour

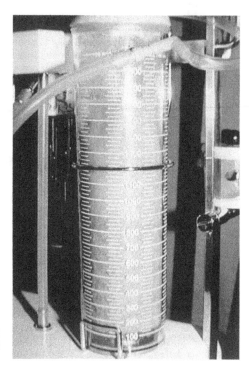

Fig. 12.12. Aspirate with only a very little blood and tumescent solution at the bottom of the column

References

1. Bonnichon P, Chapuis Y (1986) Maladie de Launois-Bensaude. Traitement par large cervico-tomie transversale. Presse Med 15:2247–2249
2. Carpeneda CA (1996) Postliposuction histologic alterations of adipose tissue. Aesth Plast Surg 20:207–211
3. Chajchir A (1996) Fat injection: long-term follow-up. Aesth Plast Surg 20:291–296
4. Coleman WP III (1988) Non-cosmetic applications of liposuction. J Dermatol Surg Oncol 14:1085–1090
5. Coleman WP III (1990) The history of liposuction. Dermatol Clin 8:381–383
6. Coleman WP III, Letessier S, Hanke CW (1997) Liposuction. In: Coleman WP III, Hanke CW, Alt TH, Asken S (eds) Cosmetic surgery of the skin, 2nd edn. Mosby, St Louis, pp 203–204
7. Dolsky RL (1990) Blood loss during liposuction. Dermatol Clin 8:463–468
8. Duskova M, Topinka H (1994) Lipomatosis benigna symmetrica. Acta Chir Plast 36:61–63
9. Feinendegen DL, Baumgartner RW, Vuadens P, Schroth G, Mattle HP, Regli F, Tschopp H (1998) Autologous fat injection for soft tissue augumentation in the face: a safe procedure? Aesth Plast Surg 22:163–167
10. Fischer A, Fischer G (1977) Revised techniques for cellulitis fat reduction in riding breeches deformity. Bull Int Acad Cosmet Surg 2:40–41
11. Goodpasture JC, Burkis J (1978) Quantitative analysis of blood and fat in suction lipectomy aspirates. Plast Reconstr Surg 78:765–772
12. Guerrerosantos J, Gonzalez-Mendoza A, Masmela Y, Gonzalez MA, Deos M, Diaz P (1996) Long-term survival of free fat grafts in muscle. An experimental study in rats. Aesth Plast Surg 20:403–408

13. Hanke CW, Bernstein G, Bullock S (1995) Safety of tumescent liposuction in 15,336 patients. Dermatol Surg 21:459–462
14. Hanke CW, Bullock S, Bernstein G (1996) Current status of tumescent liposuction in the United States. National survey results. Dermatol Surg 22:595–598
15. Illouz Y (1983) Body contouring by lipolysis: A 5 year experience with over 3000 cases. Plast Reconstr Surg 72:511–524
16. Klein JA (1987) The tumescent technique for liposuction surgery. Am J Cosm Surg 4:236–267
17. Klein JA (1990) Tumescent technique for regional anesthesia permits lidocaine doses of 35 mg/kg for liposuction., J Dermatol Surg Oncol 16:248–263
18. Klein JA (1993) Tumescent technique for regional anesthesia improves safety in large-volume liposuction. Plast Reconstr Surg 92:1085–1098
19. Klein JA (1997) The two standards of care for tumescent liposuction. Dermatol Surg 23:1194–1195
20. Lillis PJ (1988) Liposuction surgery under local anesthesia. Limited blood loss and minimal lidocaine absorption. J Dermatol Surg Oncol 14:1145–1148
21. Mevio E, Calabro P, Redaelli GA, Perano D, Rosso R (1997) Lipomatosi simmetrica benigna: malatia di Madelung. Acta Otorhinolaryngol Ital 17:64–67
22. Narins RS, Coleman WP III (1998) Minimizing pain for liposuction anesthesia. Dermatol Surg 23:1137–1140
23. Ruzicka T, Vieluf D, Landthaler M, Braun-Falco O (1987) Benign symmetric lipomatosis Launois-Bensaude. Report of ten cases and review of the literature. J Am Acad Dermatol 17:663–674
24. Sattler G, Rapprich S, Hagedorn M (1997) Tumeszenz-Lokalanästhesie- Untersuchungen zur Pharmakokinetik von Prilocain. Z Hautkr 7(72):522–525
25. Sattler G, Sommer B (1997) Liporecycling: immediate and delayed. Am J Cosm Surg 14:311–316
26. Sebastian G, Stein A, Hackert I (1998) Liposuktion zur Behandlung der benignen symmetrischen Lipomatose. Presented at the 21stAnnual Meeting of the Vereinigung für operative und onkologische Dermatologie, Kassel, 21 May1998
27. Sommer B, Sattler G (1998) Tumeszenzlokalanästhesie. Weiterentwicklung der Lokalanästhesieverfahren für die operative Dermatologie. Hautarzt 49:351–360
28. The American Society for Dermatologic Surgery (1997) Guiding principles for Liposuction. Dermatol Surg 23:1127–1129
29. Tryba M (1989) Pharmakologie und Toxikologie der Lokalanästhetika – klinische Bedeutung. Offprint from: Tryba M, Zenz M (eds) Regionalanaesthesie, 3rd edn. Gustav Fischer, Stuttgart
30. Vague J (1969) Adipo-muscular ratios in human subjects. In: Vague J, Denton R (eds) Physiopathology of adipose tissue. Excerpta Medica, Amsterdam

13 Lipomas

M. Simon

Lipomas are circumscribed, tumor-like growths of subcutaneous fat. Clinically, they usually present as subcutaneous lumps which are normally easy to move against the surrounding structures. Normally, they are covered by a thin fibrotic capsule and can then be palpated as firm, elastic, well-circumscribed tumors. Once they have reach a certain size, lipomas cause the skin to bulge out characteristically (Fig. 13.1). Subjective complaints are rare and normally occur when muscles or nerves are compressed by tumor.

On the back, neck, or shoulders, lipomas are often located subfascially or have grown together with the tough connective tissue of the skin on the back. In these cases, the typical pseudofluctuation is mostly absent and lateral mobility is significantly reduced.

Lipomas may be solitary or multiple. The occurrence of multiple lipomas in a single patient is termed "lipomatosis". There is often a genetic disposition. In other cases, lipomas are among the symptoms of complex disease manifestations (Richner–Hanhart syndrome, Gardner syndrome, neurofibromatosis, Proteus syndrome). In our experience, lipomatosis is more common in patients who are or have been intensely active in bicycling or running.

Solitary lipomas are most commonly found on the back, shoulders, hips, or on the extensor side of the thighs. Extremely large lipomas of up to 25 kg weight have been reported.

When multiple lipomas occur, they are mainly concentrated in the lower arms; they also occur in smaller numbers on the trunk and the rest of the integument.

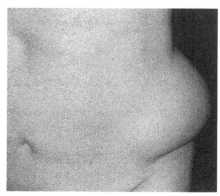

Fig. 13.1. Very large lipoma on the left flank

Lumbosacrally located lipomas are often associated with spina bifida occulta. Therefore, surgical removal of lumbosacrally located lipomas should always be preceded by further diagnostic procedures to rule out neural tube defects.

Lipomas can also be situated close to the periosteum, or may be interosseous, visceral, or inter- or intramuscular. From a technical point of view, in relation to the possibilities and limitations of TLA, the last two locations are very important, mainly because of the deep penetration and sometimes even infiltration of the striated muscles that TLA can achieve.

Special kinds of lipomas are angiolipomas, fibrolipomas, hibernomas, and some other histologic variations.

Angiolipomas are lipomas that contain a lot of blood vessels, occur mostly in young adults, and are often painful when pressure is applied. Usually, they can be differentiated macroscopically from other lipomas because of their bluish color. *Fibrolipomas* are lipomas that are filled with fibrotic structures which usually feel harder on palpation than other lipomas. Often they cannot be laterally shifted very far.

Hibernomas are very rare tumors formed of brown fetal fat. Sites of predilection are the axillas, the supraclavicular region, and the area between the shoulder blades.

Lipomas seldom become malignant. The main medical indication for surgical removal of a lipoma is therefore compression of nerves, vessels, or muscles by a tumor located at a site subject to pressure, such as the lower arm or the back, or the production of any other symptoms. Rapid progression, the exceeding of a certain size, or the presence of multiple lipomas are also indications for surgical removal. In some cases, surgical removal may be necessary for diagnostic purposes, in order to rule out other subcutaneous tumors.

In most cases, however, it is the patient who wishes to have the lipoma removed, for cosmetic reasons.

13.1 Technique

Several factors must be considered in the surgical planning. The surgical procedure depends on the size and the number of the lipomas to be removed, but the location of the growth also plays an important role in determining management:

Removal of Lipomas on the Extremities, Abdomen, and Ventral Chest Wall

Usually, the extirpation of lipomas on the extremities, the abdominal wall, and the ventral chest wall does not present any problems. Often, lipomas in these locations are easily palpable, mobile, and encapsulated. Extirpation is usually very easy by the following method:

First, the borders of the tumor as determined by palpation are marked with a skin marking pen, because palpating or otherwise making out the outlines of the lipoma is very difficult, even impossible, once TLA is established (Fig. 13.2).

After spray disinfection, a generous amount of tumescent solution is infiltrated into the subcutis in a circle around the lipoma, using a disposable cannula of suitable size with an automatic pump or else a conventional 20-ml syringe. The tip

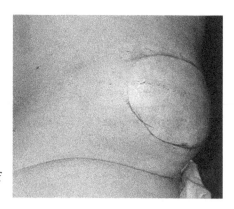

Fig. 13.2. Swollen site after infiltration of TLA and before the beginning of surgery

of the injection cannula should be directed at the base of the lipoma in order to elevate the tumor as much as possible. This technique of infiltration results in bulging firm walls of tissue abutting the lipoma, which help the expression of the tumor later on. Finally, the dermis overlying the lipoma must be infiltrated with tumescent solution in order to produce a local anesthesia that is deep enough for the incision.

After about 10 min waiting, the skin over the tumor in the skin tension lines. The lipoma capsule should be preserved if possible. The length of the incision depends on the size of the lipoma as determined earlier by palpation or ultrasonography. Usually, an incision length of about one-third of the expected tumor size is enough for easy expression of the lipoma.

Often, the lipoma has already been partly pushed through the incision by the pressure of the surrounding swollen tissue. Forceful lateral pressure applied with 2–3 fingers is usually enough to express the lipoma together with its capsule through the incision without further preparation (Fig. 13.3). With larger or more lobulated lipomas, the maneuver is usually successful after a little blunt preparation with a mosquito hemostat clamp or the surgeon's little finger.

For small lipomas, a simple skin suture followed by application of a pressure bandage is sufficient to keep the wound cavity from filling with blood and exu-

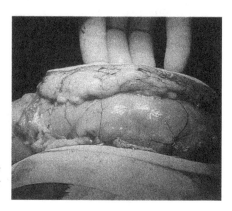

Fig. 13.3. Intraoperative finding (scale provided by the fingers of the tall senior surgeon)

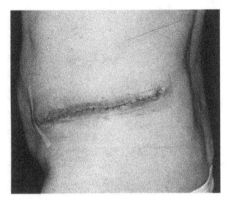

Fig. 13.4. Postoperative appearance at the first dressing change after 3 days

date. With more extensive wound cavities, it may become necessary to put in suction drainage and resect superfluous skin. After extirpation of multiple lipomas (lipomatosis), the following bandaging technique has proved effective: once the wound has been closed, the skin is brushed dry with eosin solution, then an exterior tamponade with swab balls is applied to the wound cavities and the entire extremity is wrapped in an elastic bandage (Fig. 13.4).

If the patient is compliant enough and the surgeon has the patience, a great number of lipomas can be removed by this simple method in a single session.

Removal of Lipomas of the Back and Neck

On the back and in the area of the neck, lipomas are often subfascial or have grown together with the strong connective tissue structures of the dermis. Lipomas in this location are often also filled with connective tissue septa, so that the tumors are tightly anchored to their base. For this reason, it is rarely possible to remove lipomas on the back or in the area of the neck using the simple expression technique described above.

For precise surgical planning, and to prevent any intraoperative surprises, preoperative ultrasonography of the structure to be removed is recommended. The relationship of the lipoma to its surrounding structures and its size are best assessed by scanning at 7.5 MHz.

Simple, well-circumscribed epi- or suprafascial lipomas of the back or neck region can usually be removed without problems under direct visual control after careful preparation. Preparation under direct visual control requires a significantly larger transcutaneous incision than described above.

Tumescent solution is infiltrated into the dermis and subcutis, in a circle around the lipoma being removed, as described before. Particularly with large, epifascially located lipomas, special care should be taken to ensure that the deeper layers of the subcutis and the adjacent structures have been infiltrated with enough tumescent solution, otherwise analgesia will be insufficient, particularly for preparation of the tumor base. If necessary, the base can be further infiltrated intraoperatively with 1% prilocaine solution.

Even very extended lobulated or septated lipomas on the back or in the neck areas can be removed with the same technique . Here, too, adequate analgesia at the base of the tumor is of great importance.

After the removal of large lipomas, wound closure should be done in several layers and a suction drainage inserted in order to prevent significant accumulations of exudate. Any tumescent solution that runs into the wound cavity postoperatively will also drain off this way. Any superfluous skin should be excised before final wound closure.

The application of a pressure bandage reduces the risk of postoperative complications.

Surgical removal of large subfascial or infiltrating lipomas often exceeds the limitations of TLA, since for these entities TLA alone often does not produce sufficient analgesia in the deeper layers. For small and medium-sized subfascial lipomas, however, additional intraoperative infiltration of the muscle and the epifascial connective tissue structures with 1% prilocaine solution allows operation under local anesthesia. Extended subfascial or infiltrating tumors should be removed under general anesthesia.

For large lipomas in the back or neck region, an alternative to lipoma extirpation, especially from the cosmetic point of view, is liposuction under TLA. Even for tumors in a subfascial location or with infiltrating growth, liposuction can be a real option. The suction techniques and the methods of TLA used do not differ very much from those described in Chap. 12. However, the surgeon must remember that suctioning lipomas is more difficult than suctioning normal adipose tissue, due to the presence of connective tissue cords, septae, and convoluted blood vessels.

The goal of lipoma suction is to reduce the tumor mass, so that an even skin contour can be achieved. Complete removal of the lipoma will rarely be possible with this technique, so more recurrences are to be expected than with conventional methods. In addition, to rule out the presence of an atypical lipoma or a liposarcoma, a portion of the aspirate or, better, a biopsy specimen should always be sent for histologic examination.

The advantages of liposuction are that large scars are avoided, surgery of subfascial or infiltrating lipomas is easier and less invasive, postoperative contouring is sometimes better, and occasionally several lipomas may be suctioned through one incision.

13.2 Specific Advantages

Advantages of TLA in the surgical removal of lipomas are:
- Induction of tumescent perifocal anesthesia by infiltration at the base of the lipoma allows the lipoma to be elevated and demarcated from its base.
- Because large volumes of TLA can be infiltrated, it is possible to remove virtually as many lipomas as one likes compared to what can be done with traditional methods of local anesthesia. At our institution, for example, a patient with familial lipomatosis had 147 lipomas expressed in one session (Figs. 13.5, 13.6).

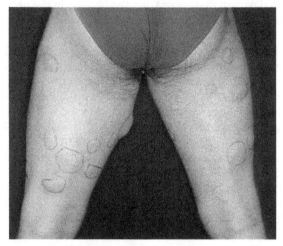

Fig. 13.5. Patient with multiple lipomas of the extremities

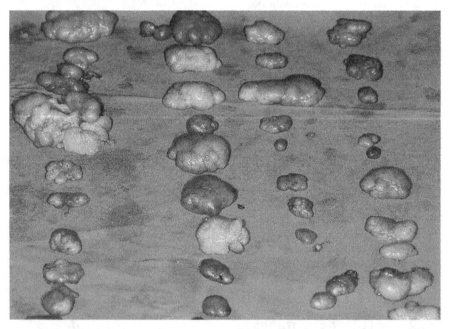

Fig. 13.6. Multiple lipomas. These are some of the 147 lipomas removed in one session under TLA

- The vasoconstrictive effects of the added epinephrine and the vasocompression resulting from the volume of infiltrated tumescent solution mean that most lipomas can be removed almost without loss of blood.
- If hematomas do nevertheless occur, the diluting effect of the infiltrated tumescent solution allows them to be better resorbed, while at the same time the solution's antibacterial effect also helps to prevent infections.

- Even very large lipomas can usually be removed under TLA without any problems. Alternatively, techniques of liposuction under TLA can also be employed.
- The slow infiltration and marked lipophilia of prilocaine together with the effects of the added vasoconstrictors mean that TLA has a long-lasting action that renders postoperative pain medication virtually unnecessary.

13.3 Specific Disadvantages

Disadvantages of TLA in the surgical removal of lipomas are:
- Palpation and delimitation of the lipoma after a long TLA anesthesia time is very difficult, even impossible.
- If tumescent solution is inadvertently infiltrated into the lipoma, the latter may swell up, making extirpation more difficult.

References

1. Braun-Falco O, Plewig G, Wolff HH (1995) Dermatologie und Venerologie. 4th edn. Springer, Berlin Heidelberg New York Tokyo
2. Coleman WP (1988) Non-cosmetic applications of liposuction. J Dermatol Surg Oncol 14:1085–1090
3. Harrington AC, Adnot J, Chesser RS (1990) Infiltrating lipomas of the upper extremities. J Dermatol Surg Oncol 16:834–837
4. Kenawi MM (1995) "Squeeze delivery" excision of subcutaneous lipoma related to anatomic site. Br J Surg 82:1649–1650
5. Leffell DJ, Braverman IM (1986) Familial multiple lipomatosis. Report of a case and a review of the literature. J Am Acad Dermatol 15:275–279
6. Nichter LS, Gupta BR (1990) Liposuction of giant lipoma. Ann Plast Surg 24: 362–365
7. Orfanos CE, Garbe C (1995) Therapie der Hautkrankheiten, 1st edn. Springer, Berlin Heidelberg New York Tokyo
8. Pinski KS, Roenigk HH Jr (1990) Liposuction of lipomas. Dermatol Clin 8: 483–492
9. Sanchez MR, Golomb FM, Moy JA, Potozkin JR (1993) Giant lipoma: case report and review of the literature. J Am Acad Dermatol 28: 266–268
10. Sommer B, Sattler G (1998) Tumeszenzlokalanästhesie. Weiterentwicklung der Lokalanästhesieverfahren für die operative Dermatologie. Hautarzt 49: 351–360
11. Wihelm KP, Eisenbeiss W, Wolff HH (1993) Hibernom der Stirn. Hautarzt 44: 735–737

14 Large Excisions

B. Sommer, D. Bergfeld

The two most recent – and outstanding – German standard works on surgical dermatology do not yet mention tumescent technique [4, 5]. In this chapter we will show that large excisions do not necessarily require general anesthesia, as is claimed in these works [6].

Theoretically, almost any skin lesion can be treated under TLA. Naturally, individual factors must be taken into account, such as the patient's anxiety level and the nature of surgery (see also Chap. 11). Under general anesthesia procedures can be extended in area without worrying about how far, whereas intraoperative changes in surgery performed under local anesthesia require further injection of TLA solution. If the patient suffers pain or moves about in a way that causes problems during surgery under general anesthesia, that is the business of the anesthesiologist. With TLA, the adequacy of anesthesia is the surgeon's responsibility. In most cases, though, the possibility of large-scale local anesthesia is a blessing for both patient and surgeon: reduced bleeding makes operating easier, while perfect postoperative mobilization, reduced pain, and improved healing speed up convalescence. Thus, extensive procedures can be performed on an outpatient basis or with a much shorter hospital stay, and, finally, costs are reduced.

Anecdotally, we would like to mention that at our institution many surgeons had difficulty in getting used to the procedure and the advantages of TLA. Early on, therefore, despite the existing reports in literature [2], the incision line was infiltrated additionally with the familiar 1% lidocaine or prilocaine, owing to remaining doubts about the anesthetic potency of the TLA solution.

Our experiences, especially those relating to the injection technique, are presented below.

14.1 Technique

Once the planned incision line has been precisely marked, 1% local anesthetic (prilocaine) is injected to form individual intracutaneous wheals into which the TLA is infiltrated. These should follow the planned incision line.

Using a 25-gauge cannula and a manual or an electrical pump, a 0.05–0.1% TLA solution containing prilocaine is slowly infiltrated subcutaneously into the wheals. Depending on the need for subcutaneous mobilization, the surrounding tissue is also infiltrated.

If a hard tissue turgor is desired, the planned incision line should be additionally infiltrated just subcutaneously or even intracutaneously with 1% local anesthetic, since it takes about 10 min until complete anesthesia is reached using only TLA.

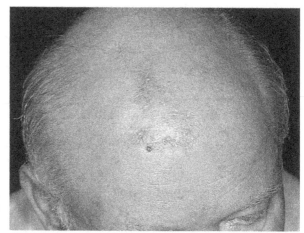

Fig. 14.1. Large frontal morphea-like basal cell carcinoma

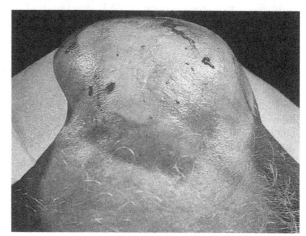

Fig. 14.2. Large swelling = tumescence after the infiltration. The longer one waits, the greater the "mini-expander" effect

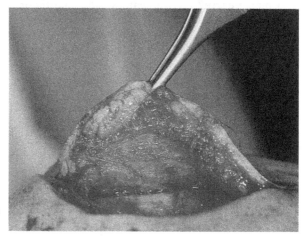

Fig. 14.3. Starting excision under TLA

If the tissue turgor is a minor concern, one can wait with the incision for about 15–20 min, and the additional injection with 1% local anesthetic becomes unnecessary.

The infusion of large volumes of TLA, and repeat infusion when tissue turgor decreases, allows the TLA solution to be used as a short-term expander (Fig. 14.1, 14.2).

If, on the other hand, the excision is to be followed by immediate primary wound margin approximation, one must make sure not to infuse too much TLA solution, because this can make primary wound closure more difficult. To distinguish it from the almost watermelon-like consistency that is desirable for liposuction procedures, we call this kind of infiltration technique "semi-tumescence," because the turgor at the end of infusion is much softer.

14.2 Specific Advantages

The "bloodlessness" of the tissue preparation in TLA, due to the epinephrine additive, is impressive. The subcutaneous structures are stretched by the infused fluid, facilitating the excision [1]. This effect is also known as hydrodissection and from the surgical point of view is an entirely desirable feature of TLA.

As already mentioned in other chapters, the patient benefits from a prolonged pain-free period, very low bleeding – and thus a reduced incidence of postoperative hematomas – and more rapid postoperative mobilization [3,7].

Although the surgical site is somewhat wetter with TLA than in an operation performed under general anesthesia, the vasoconstriction caused by the epinephrine additive in the TLA solution, together with the atraumatic preparation technique, leads to significantly less intraoperative bleeding (Fig. 14.3), which improves the surgeon's view of the operative site and makes the surgery easier [1]. After preparation is complete, meticulous hemostasis is nevertheless necessary even though bleeding is only slight, because bleeding could still start later as the vasoconstrictor effect wears off.

At the end of surgery, wound closure is carried out with subcutaneous sutures followed by skin sutures (any suturing techniques may be used).

The advantages of TLA for large excisions are:

Complete freedom from pain without anesthetic risk.
- Hydrodissection effect of TLA; atraumatic surgical procedure.
- Little intraoperative bleeding because of the vasoconstrictive effect of TLA.
- Active movement is possible during wound closure, so any misalignment can be corrected intraoperatively.
- Pre-expanding ("mini-expander") effect of TLA.
- Long-lasting postoperative analgesia.

14.3 Specific Disadvantages

The disadvantages of TLA for large excisions are:
- Meticulous surgical planning is necessary, since the skin tension lines and the tumor margins are unrecognizable after infiltration.
- Sources of bleeding are harder to identify.

- There is increased postoperative swelling.
- Wound closure is performed under relatively high skin tension.

References

1. Acosta AE (1997) Clinical parameters of tumescent anesthesia in skin cancer reconstructive surgery. A review of 86 patients. Arch Dermatol 133: 451–454
2. Coleman WP, Klein JA (1992) Use of the tumescent technique for scalp surgery, dermabrasion, and soft tissue reconstruction. J Dermatol Surg Oncol 18: 130–135
3. Kalodikis L, Hermes B, Kohl PK (1998) Tumeszenz-Lokalanästhesie. Einsatz im Kopfbereich. Z Hautkr 73: 316–317
4. Kaufmann R, Landes E (1992) Dermatologische Operationen. Farbatlas und Lehrbuch der Hautchirurgie, 2nd edn. Thieme, Stuttgart New York
5. Petres J, Rompel R (1996) Operative Dermatologie. Lehrbuch und Atlas. Springer, Berlin Heidelberg New York Tokyo
6. Petres J, Rompel R (1996) Regionale operative Verfahren, Stamm. In: Petres J, Rompel R (eds) Operative Dermatologie. Lehrbuch und Atlas. Springer, Berlin Heidelberg New York Tokyo, pp 371–452
7. Sattler G (1998) Lokalanästhesie, Regionalanästhesie, Tumeszenzanästhesie: Techniken und Indikationen. Z Hautkr 73:316

15 Abdominoplasty

B. BLUGERMAN, D. SCHAVELZON

Only in exceptional cases is surgical tightening of the abdominal wall performed for functional reasons. Usually, it is a cosmetic procedure. Which surgical method is chosen depends on the underlying fat deformity. Where there is localized fat proliferation beneath a firm, elastic abdominal wall, liposuction is the method of choice. In cases where the skin has become markedly slack or genuinely superfluous skin is present, abdominoplasty should be considered [2].

The use of new suction cannulas has in fact reduced the number of cases in which surgical tightening of the abdominal wall is necessary, since connective tissue structures are now to a large extent preserved and therefore good skin retraction may be expected. This is why abdominoplasty is nowadays indicated only in rare cases [3].

In all cases, the fat depot should first be reduced by means of liposuction, because this reduces the weight pulling downward on the skin. In addition, it is known that liposuction and the resulting trauma induce a diffuse fibrosis which stabilizes the remaining subcutaneous fat [1]. If an abdominoplasty is carried out later, this fat stabilization will make it easier. If both procedures are performed in one session, the increased complication rate must be taken into account.

In our experience the concentration of the normal Klein solution is inadequate. The mixture shown in Table 15.1 has worked well for us over the past years.

The infiltration of tumescent solution has three main functions to perform:
- Adequate anesthesia
- Hydrodissection
- Good hemostasis.

Table 15.1. Recipe for approx. 0.15% tumescent solution

Isotonic saline solution	1000 ml
Lidocaine 2% with epinephrine 1/100 000	80 ml[a]
Sodium bicarbonate 8.4%	40 ml
Epinephrine 1:1000	1 ml

[a] *Editors' note:* At the present time clinical studies exist only for 0.05% TLA solution and clinical experiences only for TLA solutions of 0.1% or less. It should be noted, even though clinical experience differs sharply from this, that the manufacturer's recommended maximum dose of lidocaine is 10 ml in a 2% solution.

15.1 Technique

Before infusion starts, the planned incision line and the surgical site are precisely marked out. A seemingly trivial point is correct choice and use of the marking pen, since, especially in TLA, there is always a lot of fluid in the surgical field, which can wash away the markings. We always add vertical lines, which make it easier to identify corresponding structures during wound closure.

After the wheals of local anesthetic have been injected, infusion of standard TLA solution is begun (see Chap. 9). The aim is to induce a not too hard turgor. If tumescence is insufficient, full anesthesia may not be achieved and vasoconstriction is inadequate; but, on the other hand, if tumescence is too hard, the surgical site contains a very great deal of fluid, and it can be difficult to approximate the wound margins without tension. In case of doubt, too much tumescence is better than too little. On average, 4000–7000 ml tumescent solution is needed for this.

The superficial infusion can be performed with the afore-mentioned 20-gauge cannula. At 7 cm it is not always long enough, however, so for larger fat accumulations the multiple-hole cannula (e.g., infusion needles from Wells Johnson Co., see Appendix C) is more suitable. Such infusion needles are available with one or more holes down the side of the cannula, through which the TLA solution is poured into the subcutaneous fat as from a watering can. Standard diameters are 1.5, 2.0, and 3.0 mm in variable lengths from 10 to 40 cm.

Anesthesia waiting time should be at least 10 min in order to make full use of the anesthetic and vasoconstrictive effects. If it is desirable to begin surgery earlier, 1% local anesthetic can be injected along the incision lines. Alternatively the tumescent solution can be used for a very superficial infusion resulting in the so called "peau d'orange" effect. There are many more free nerve endings available for nociception in the dermis than in the subcutis, and for this reason painfree surgery can be carried out in the subcutaneous tissue before the dermis has lost all sensitivity. This can be circumvented by the above-mentioned additional infusion of normal-concentration local anesthetic.

It is sensible to keep the tumescent solution within reach in case areas are found during surgery that are still sensitive or have been insufficiently infiltrated.

Determining factors in the surgical planning include not only the nature of the fat deformity, but also the desired location of the scar (which requires preoperative marking of the swimsuit lines).

In cases where a combined liposuction and skin resection is necessary, we do the liposuction first in order to find remaining stable tissue. This also avoids the problem of tumescent solution leaking from the incision lines.

In combined procedures the retraction of the skin induced by the liposuction must be factored in, meaning that the area of skin marked for resection should be slightly smaller than in traditional abdominoplasties. In this way, scar contraction, hypertrophic and keloid scars, and misalignments of skin over prominent places can be avoided.

If the straight abdominal muscle is to be sutured during the abdominoplasty, we infiltrate the tumescent solution through a small opening directly beneath the aponeurosis of the muscle. This prevents pain arising from the pulling and suturing on the aponeurosis.

The standard procedure starts with the lower incision in the groin, continuing with blunt preparation of the fat cushion on the lateral side and sharp preparation medially, cutting it from the muscle fascia. Meticulous hemostasis of the epigastric and the many perforating blood vessels is mandatory.

We like to use the electrical monopolar blade, since the electrocoagulation ensures good hemostasis.

After preparation up to the navel, the navel is "freed" from the sorrounding skin, and the remaining tissue is then mobilized up to the lowest rib. Medially above the navel there is often a dense net of fibers passing through the fat which makes it necessary to cut the fat from the fascia. Laterally, blunt preparation is easy.

After complete mobilization up to the lowest rib and the xiphoid, the prepared flap is gently pulled down. The aim is to ensure approximation of the wound margins under as little tension as possible. If necessary and if there has been no prior liposuction, one can use a blade to thin out the subcutaneous tissue of the upper abdominal flap along the scarpas fascia. Any other fat corrections necessary can be performed now, e.g., resection or suction of lateral or lumbar fat cushions or suction of the medial aspect of the thighs. All these can be performed from the inguinal wound margin.

After reimplantation of the navel, wound margin approximation is usually performed with a continuous subcutaneous suture in combination with a continuous intracutaneous suture.

Depending on the primary findings, there are several variations to the standard procedure described here, e.g., upper and lower abdominoplasty.

15.2   Specific Advantages

Currently, TLA is mostly used by dermatologists, but it is also starting to make its way into plastic surgery. In our practice more than 90% of all procedures are performed under TLA. Other abdominal procedures to be mentioned include dermalipectomy (conventional with navel transposition and en bloc with neoumbilicoplasty), minidermolipectomy (conventional and endoscopic), lumbar plasty, and scar revision. A few reports have now been published by surgeons supporting our positive experiences [4].

Advantages of TLA in abdominoplasty are:
- Only minimal sedation is necessary.
- Safe anesthesia without the risks of general anesthesia.
- Easy separation of layers due to the prepreparation/hydrodissection effect.
- Reduced bleeding means a clear operative field.
- A combined procedure with liposuction is possible.
- Low postoperative hematoma rate.
- Patient recovery is more rapid.
- Low thrombosis risk.

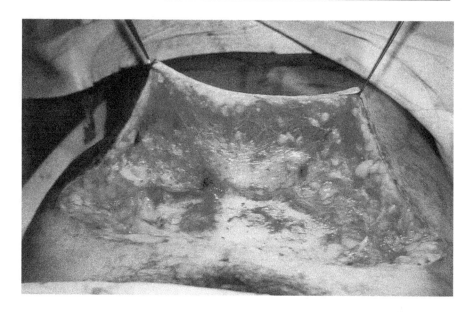

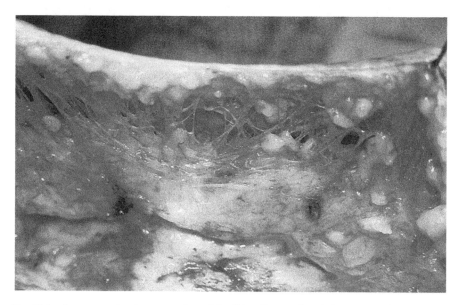

Fig. 15.1. Intraoperative demonstration of the "bloodlessness" and the preserved connective tissue and blood vessels after liposuction and during the abdominoplasty

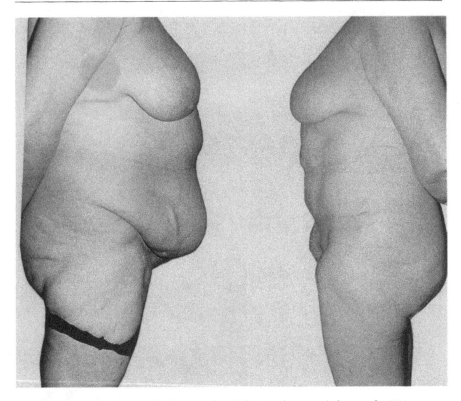

Fig. 15.2. Pre- and postoperative images of an abdominoplasty carried out under TLA

15.3 Specific Disadvantages

Disadvantages of TLA in abdominoplasty are:
- Higher incidence of seromas or serosanguinous collections.
- Hemostasis is slightly more difficult due to the large fluid volumes, with result-ant risk of postoperative bleeding.
- Preoperative markings may be washed off.
- Postoperative leaking of tumescent solution.
- Reduced adherence of adhesive dressings.

References

1. Carpeneda CA (1996) Postliposuction histologic alterations of adipose tissue. Aesth Plast Surg 20: 207–211
2. Kesselring UK (1998) Die Bauchdeckenstraffung. In: Lemperle G (eds) Aesthetische Chirurgie. Ecomed, Landsberg, pp X1-X11
3. Matarasso A, Matarasso S (1998) When does your liposuction patient require an abdomino-plasty? Dermatol Surg 23: 1151–1160
4. Nguyen TT, Kim KA, Young RB (1997) Tumescent mini abdominoplasty. Ann Plast Surg 38: 209–212

16 Medial Thigh Lift

G. SATTLER, B. SOMMER

The skin and the subcutaneous connective and supportive tissues on the medial side of the adult female thigh are especially soft. In addition, depending on predisposition, there are fat accumulations of varying sizes and experienced as disturbing to varying degrees. The combination of these factors can lead to the so-called "stage curtain phenomenon", dermatochalasis of the inner aspects of the thighs.

As a general rule, liposuction is performed first to remove the excessive fat. This relieves the skin of the weight of the fat pulling it down under gravity. Overall, the medial aspects of the thighs show a only moderate tendency to retract (see Chap. 12), so that where dermatochalasis is advanced a medial thigh lift is indicated. Within certain limits, the skin can be pulled tight during this, but patients should be warned not to raise their hopes too high as to how long the result will last.

16.1 Technique

Basically, the skin is resected so that adaptation to external rotation is still possible. The size of the skin flap to be resected is determined properatively with the patient standing upright.

Overcorrection should be avoided for several reasons. For one thing, strong pulling can cause dehiscences, which will later retract. What should be remembered is that the reduction in skin elasticity itself cannot be treated, only the effects it is having currently. Strong pulling will therefore only lead to even faster stretching of the skin, endangering the overall result. There is also a risk of distorting the labia majora.

Once the skin wheals are injected with 1% local anesthetic, infusion can begin. The tissue turgor aimed at is less than desired for liposuction procedures; on palpation the incompletely swollen subcutaneous fat should feel something like a half-inflated air mattress. Induction of normal tumescence may hinder tension-free wound closure at the end of the procedure. If normal tumescent solution is used, the epinephrine additive provides for sufficient vasoconstriction.

The incision line runs from the inguinal crease arteriorly to the infragluteal crease posteriorly; distally, a half-moon-shaped skin flap is resected, the size of which depends on the primary findings. It is important to attach the skin of the thigh to the periosteum of the pubis and ischium with strong subcutaneous sutures in order to prevent the weight of the skin from causing dehiscence or pulling on the labia majora. The skin is closed with a skin suture or tacking.

After application of a compression bandage or a common compression stocking, the patient is mobilized immediately postoperatively.

16.2   Specific Advantages

Advantages of TLA in medial thigh lift are:
- Only minimal sedation is necessary.
- Safe anesthesia without the risks of general anesthesia.
- Prepreparation/hydrodissection effect.
- Reduced bleeding results in a clear operative field.
- Low postoperative hematoma rate.
- Rapid patient recovery.
- Low risk of thrombosis.

16.3   Specific Disadvantages

Disadvantages of TLA in medial thigh lift are:
- Postoperative leaking of tumescent fluid.
- Wound margin approximation is difficult, especially if too much TLA solution has been infused.

References

1. Kesselring U (1998) Oberschenkelstraffung. In: Lemperle G (eds) Aesthetische Chirurgie. Ecomed, Landsberg, pp XI-3 1–5
2. Schultz RC, Feinber LA (1979) Medial thigh lift. Ann Plast Surg 2: 404–410

17 Tumescent Facelift

D. Spencer, C.W. Hanke

17.1 Technique

Recommended Tumescent Solution

Correct preparation of the tumescent solution for a facelift is essential for the safety and comfort of the patient. The appropriate mixture for this procedure contains 0.1% lidocaine (100 ml 1% lidocaine per 1000 ml physiological saline), epinephrine 1:250,000 (4 ml 1:1000 epinephrine per 1000 ml physiological saline), and 20 ml sodium bicarbonate. In addition, some surgeons like to add triamcinolone 10 mg per 1000 ml physiological saline in order to reduce the postoperative tendency to swelling.

Preoperative Preparation

The patient's medical and psychological history are taken, preoperative laboratory results are reviewed, and informed consent is obtained. Prophylactic antibiotic treatment (cephalexin 500 mg b.i.d) is started on the morning of surgery and continued for 7 days. The face and neck areas are washed with an antibacterial soap (e.g., Dial or Lever 2000) the evening before and the morning of surgery. The patient is transported to the surgical suite and is prepared routinely. The planned areas for facelift and neck liposuction are outlined with a marking pen. The hair in the temporal area and postauricular/mastoid area is secured with tape or barrettes. Some patients receive preoperative sedation (promethazine 25 mg i.m., meperidine 50 mg i.m., and midazolam 5 mg i.m.). Most patients, however, are content to do without sedation once they are adequately informed about the benefits of TLA.

Operative Technique

Heart rate, cardiac rhythm, and oxygen saturation are monitored continuously during the neck liposuction and facelift. The patient is positioned upright and the relevant skin area prepped with Phisoderm. Infusion of tumescent solution into the neck and postauricular sulci is begun via the usual infusion cannulas. Three 3.0-mm-long incisions are then made in these three areas with a no. 11 blade, and tumescent solution injected into the facial area through these incisions using a Hunstad Autofuse handle (Fig. 17.1). In this instrument, a 12-gauge infusion cannula

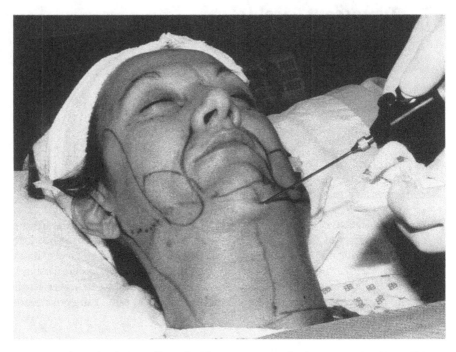

Fig. 17.1. The neck is being infiltrated with tumescent anesthesia. Preoperative skin markings are present

connects the handpiece to a 1-l bag of tumescent solution which is surrounded by a pressure cuff. Other infusion methods can be utilized, including electrical pumps (Wells Johnson Co. or Byron Medical, see Appendix C).

In order to minimize patient discomfort, the tumescent solution is instilled slowly, beginning with the neck region and then moving to the preauricular planes. As infiltration of each new plane starts, the patient may experience a slight burning sensation, but the discomfort lasts only a few seconds and can be reduced by allowing the solution to dissect ahead of the infusion cannula.

In women, generally 750 ml tumescent solution is required for the face and neck and 200 ml for each side of the face. In men, 1 l solution is needed for the face and neck and 250 ml for each side of the face. Infusion lasts approximately 15 min: 5 min for the neck and 5 min for each side of the face. The tumescent solution causes vasoconstriction, leading to the appearance of a blanching effect about 15 min after infusion starts.

Liposuction of the neck is performed in the usual fashion with a microcannula. A 12-gauge microcannula with a 2.0-mm internal diameter is preferred to a 14-gauge cannula because the latter may bend and even break. Following liposuction of the neck, platysmal bands are repaired with 3–0 Mersilene sutures.

The facelift operation proper proceeds with undermining and mobilization of the skin using Metzenbaum scissors, starting from the same 3.0 mm incisions previously utilized for infusion of tumescent solution. The preparation plane is

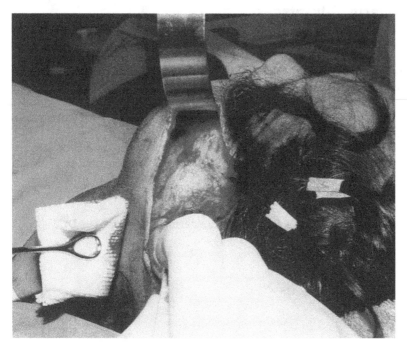

Fig. 17.2.   Tumescent anesthesia allows the SMAS to be visualized with very little bleeding

3–5 mm below the skin in the subcutaneous fat. This plane, above the superficial muscular aponeurotic system (SMAS), is chosen in order not to damage branches of the facial nerve. After undermining is complete, a continuous incision is made extending from the temporal hairline to the post-tragal area (or pretragal if necessary), postauricular sulcus, and masto-occipital area. This is followed by preauricular and postauricular undermining and electrodessication of bleeding vessels – although bleeding vessels are rare in facelifts performed under TLA (Fig. 17.2). The SMAS is plicated using four to six permanent Mersilene sutures. Any remaining fat lobules are trimmed away with the Metzenbaum scissors and excess skin in the temporal, preauricular, and masto-occipital areas is trimmed. This may amount to 1.0–2.0 cm for the anterior flap and 0.5–1.0 cm for the posterior flap. The skin edges are approximated using interlocking, continuous 5-o silk in front of the ear and 3-o silk behind the ear. The temporal and masto-occipital skin is approximated with staples.

The total length of time for the whole procedure is 2.5–3.0 h.

A face/neck dressing is placed over the neck and lateral face. We use cotton and Coban for this (3M Pharmaceuticals, see Appendix C). The dressing absorbs any oozing of the tumescent solution that may occur.

Most tumescent facelift patients have very little postoperative discomfort. Ecchymosis resolves in 7–10 days. Bruising is minimal compared to conventional nontumescent facelift.

17.2   Specific Advantages

Specific advantages of TLA for facelift are:
- The risks and added expense of general anesthesia are eliminated.
- Postoperative nausea and vomiting are minimized because of the absence of general anesthesia.
- Tumescent anesthesia has allowed facelifting to be performed totally under local anesthesia with less bleeding and more rapid postoperative recovery than in conventional facelift.
  - The aesthetic result of tumescent facelift is comparable to that of conventional facelift. Patients who have experienced both conventional "dry" facelift and tumescent facelift prefer the latter procedure over the former.

This chapter is dedicated to a great American dermatologist, the late Dr. Malcolm C. Spencer, who passed away in January 1998.

18   Skin Flaps

S. SATTLER

Until a couple of years ago, extensive skin flaps, especially in skin tumor surgery, had to be performed under general anesthesia. Because of the toxicologic properties of commercially available local anesthetics, the amounts needed exceeded the maximum dose. Therefore, dermatologists and maxillofacial and plastic surgeons were dependent on anesthesiologic support. The patient usually had to be hospitalized for a few days.

Since the introduction of TLA, it has been possible to perform these procedures on an outpatient basis safely and without a lot of equipment. In addition, some technical aspects of the surgery are made easier by the tumescent solution, as will be described below. Basically, all forms of skin flap surgery can be performed under TLA [2, 3].

18.1   Technique

After precise marking of the planned incision line, intracutaneous wheals of 1% local anesthetic (prilocaine) are injected, into which the TLA is infused. It is advisable to place them along the planned incision line.

A 0.05%–0.1% TLA solution of prilocaine is infiltrated subcutaneously into the wheals with a 25-gauge needle and a manual infusion pump or an electrical pump set at a slow rate. The infiltration area should include the entire surgical site. In addition to the planned incision line, all the surrounding subcutaneous tissue needed for the mobilization of the skin flap should be infiltrated (Fig. 18.1).

Compared to the use of TLA in liposuction, the infiltration here should be so moderate that the advantages of the solution itself (complete anesthesia, vasoconstriction, mobilization) can be exploited. If the tissue tension gets too high, wound closure will be inhibited later on. After a short anesthesia waiting time (a couple of minutes), surgery can commence.

The main points of the surgical procedure are:
- Surgical planning, patient information, patient consent
- Photo documentation
- Intravenous catheter
- Marking of the incision line
- Injection of subcutaneous wheals with 1% local anesthetic (e.g., prilocaine)
- Infiltration of the TLA (0.05% prilocaine), *moderate* tumescence!
- Atraumatic flap preparation
- Meticulous hemostasis
- Wound closure.

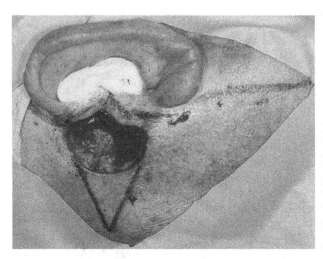

Fig. 18.1. Appearance after removal of a preauricular basal cell carcinoma. Wound closure is planned with a double skin flap after three-dimensional histological wound margin study. The photograph was taken after subcutaneous infiltration of TLA

18.2   Specific Advantages

In the preparation of skin flaps under TLA, what is striking is how easy it is to separate the subcutaneous structures from each other – almost entirely by blunt dissection. This is due to the tumescent solution which flows around the connective tissue septae, thus separating the subcutaneous tissue (fat). The process may be called hydrodissection. Thanks to this prepreparation effect of TLA, tissue is damaged a lot less, and important structures (vessels and nerves) can be easily prepared without risk. Even for smaller skin flap procedures, the tumescent hydrodissection effect is superior to ordinary local anesthesia because of the lower risk of intravenous or intramuscular administration.

Although the surgical site is overall somewhat wetter with TLA than in an operation performed under general anesthesia, the epinephrine additive in the solution causes vasoconstriction. This, together with the atraumatic preparation technique, results in significantly less intraoperative bleeding (Fig. 18.2), giving a better surgical view and facilitating the operation [1]. At the end of the preparation, meticulous hemostasis is necessary even though bleeding is slight, because otherwise postoperative bleeding may occur as the vasoconstrictor effect wears off.

At the end of surgery, wound closure is accomplished with a subcutaneous suture followed by a skin suture (all suture techniques are applicable) (Fig. 18.3). Especially in operations in the facial area, the patient can make all the relevant movements during wound closure (unlike operations under general anesthesia), so that any distortion caused by the surgery can be recognized intraoperatively and can be corrected in the same session.

Advantages of TLA in skin flap surgery are:

- Complete freedom from pain without the risks associated with general anesthesia.
- Hydrodissection effect of TLA, atraumatic surgical procedure.

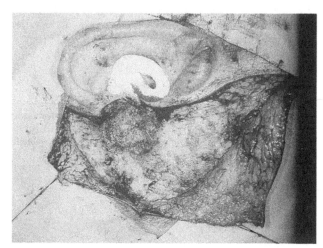

Fig. 18.2. Intraoperative photograph during the skin flap preparation

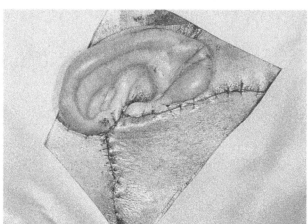

Fig. 18.3. Wound margin approximation is complete

- Little intraoperative bleeding because of vasoconstrictive effect of TLA.
- Facial movements possible during wound closure, so any misalignment can be corrected intraoperatively.
- Flap is protected from desiccation during surgery.
- "Mini-expander" effect of TLA.
- Long-lasting postoperative analgesia.

Disadvantages of TLA in skin flap surgery are:
- Precise surgical planning is necessary, since tumor margins are unrecognizable after infiltration.
- Skin tension lines are unrecognizable after infiltration.
- Identifying the sources of bleeding is more difficult.
- Wound closure takes place under relatively high skin tension.
- Intraoperative and postoperative swelling are increased.

Evaluation of Indication: Skin flap surgery is well suited for TLA.

Recommended TLA Concentration: 0.1%–0.2% in the head area, 0.1%–0.5% in the trunk and extremities.

References

1. Acosta AE (1997) Clinical parameters of tumescent anesthesia in skin cancer reconstructive surgery. A review of 86 patients. Arch Dermatol 133: 451–454
2. Kalodikis L, Hermes B, Kohl PK (1998) Tumeszenz-Lokalanästhesie. Einsatz im Kopfbereich. Z Hautkr 73: 316–317
3. Sattler G (1998) Lokalanästhesie, Regionalanästhesie, Tumeszenzanästhesie: Techniken und Indikationen. Z Hautkr 73: 316

19   Split-Thickness Grafts

B. SOMMER

If the size of the surgical site makes primary closure or closure with a skin flap impossible, free transplantation is indicated. Usually, after extended local excision of melanomas and after waiting for wound granulation, wound defects are covered with split-thickness grafts; extended ulcers of the lower leg are covered with split-thickness skin, especially after derma-shaving therapy.

Split-thickness grafts consist of epidermis and dermis and are classified according to their thickness into thin (£0.3 mm), intermediate (0.4–0.5 mm), and thick (about 0.6 mm) transplants. The excision is performed with a dermatome; the depth and width of the transplant can be variably adjusted. The dermatome must be firmly applied to the skin and pushed slowly forward because the freshly excised transplant may otherwise be in danger of getting caught in the dermatome blade again. The transplants can be meshed either by hand or, more evenly, by a mechanical dermatome ("mesh graft") [2].

19.1   Technique

The TLA solution can be infused in different ways.

Disposable Cannulas

The TLA solution can be infused like an ordinary local anesthetic using a 20-gauge disposable cannula (0.9 mm diameter) and 10 ml- or 20 ml- syringes, depending on the size of the area to be infiltrated. It is important to place the cannula just beneath the dermis. If a larger area is to be injected, it is best to use a 7-cm-long version of the 20-gauge cannula, since this means that the skin is punctured less often.

Pseudotumescent Solution

If the area to be infiltrated is not extensive, and there is no pre-mixed TLA at hand, it is not necessary to prepare a new solution for such a small procedure. In such cases, the surgeon can mix a "pseudotumescent solution" by drawing lidocaine or prilocaine with an epinephrine additive into a 20-ml-syringe up to the 5- to 10-ml mark (depending on the desired onset of effect: the lower the concentration

of the local anesthetic, the later it starts to act). One can then draw up
1–2 ml of sodium bicarbonate into the same syringe; the remaining volume is then
filled with physiological saline or Ringer's solution (see Chap. 9). This procedure
can be repeated once if the volume of the solution is insufficient. The technique
is worthwhile and recommended only if the area to be anesthetized is too extensive for a conventional local anesthetic, but not so extensive that it requires using a 500-ml bottle. Also, the proportion of local anesthetic used in this method
is higher than in the usual TLA solutions, and there is a danger of adverse effects
if solution mixed in this way is given in large volumes.

Blunt Infiltration Cannulas

For the infiltration of the donor area, a blunt infusion cannula of the kind used
for the anesthesia of certain areas in abdominal liposuction is used [1]. This kind
of infusion cannula is manufactured by the following companies (see Appendix
C): Tulip, a 5-hole cannula (Tulip Company, San Diego, California, USA) or Klein's
"multiple-hole infusion needles", best in a diameter of 1.5 or 2 mm (Wells Johnson
Co.). The last named are avaible in the standard lengths of 10 cm, 15 cm, and 20 cm.
"Three-hole spatula-type infusion needles for facial procedures" are also available, and are equally suitable.

The sites for the small stab incisions into which the cannulas are inserted are
first injected with wheals of local anesthetic. The cannula is then inserted up subcutaneously to the furthest point that is to be anesthetized. As it is pulled back,
TLA solution is infiltrated into the tissue from a bag or syringe until a "peau
d'orange" effect occurs. The whole area is then similarly anesthetized in a fan-
shaped fashion; if necessary, more stab incisions can be made on opposing sides.

19.2 Specific Advantages

As already mentioned, even extensive areas can be anesthetized comfortably and
very safely with the tumescent method.

An immeasurable advantage in the split-thickness graft excision is the good
passive resistance provided by the bulging tissue turgor in a correctly performed
TLA. For this reason, it is important to make sure that not too much time passes
between the infusion and the procedure, since the turgor gradually diminishes by
diffusion of the fluid into the surrounding tissue. Tightening the skin to facilitate
the procedure is not necessary with TLA, so one can concentrate totally on harvesting the split-thickness graft from the moving dermatome.

Because the subcutaneous tissue is equally tumescent everywhere, the split-
thickness graft being harvested can be kept equally thick in all parts, even in difficult areas, e.g., gluteally, or in older people whose skin is especially loose or who
have irregular skin in the thigh area due to senile atrophy.

Bleeding is minimal, owing to the already described effects of the epinephrine
additive and the blood vessel compression – something that also makes applying the dressings easier.

In our experience, wound healing is more rapid than with common methods; however, this phenomenon has not yet been proven in clinical studies.

Specific advantages in split-thickness graft transplantation are:
- Comfortable anesthesia even of extensive areas
- Good passive resistance for harvesting the split-thickness graft
- Minimal bleeding
- Good wound healing at the harvest site.

References

1. Field LM, Hrabovszy T (1997) Harvesting split-thickness grafts with tumescent anesthesia. Letter to the editor. Dermatol Surg 23:62
2. Kaufmann R, Landes E (1992) Dermatologische Operationen, 2nd edn. Thieme, Stuttgart New York, pp 56 ff

20 Dermabrasion

A. Picoto

During a visit to our center in Lisbon in 1994, Dr. Lawrence Field demonstrated the use of Klein's tumescent local anesthesia in large skin flaps in the facial area. We found the low incidence of bleeding and hematomas together with the increased ease of tissue preparation with this method very persuasive.

We soon got the idea of utilizing it for full-face-dermabrasions for correction of acne scars. Since then it has become our routine method of anesthesia for this procedure, sometimes in combination with regional nerve blocks. Later, we discovered that Coleman and Klein had already described the use of TLA for dermabrasion in 1992 [1].

Dermabrasion can be used to correct uneven skin or to ablate or remove skin alterations or foreign bodies [5]. Today, for many indications the primary technique is careful abrading of the skin by experienced surgeons with a diamond fraise. Among the indications are correction of acne scars, ablation of syringomas, treatment of perioral wrinkles, removal of seborrheic keratoses or wide-spread lentigines simplex. Until now, the treatment of large skin areas was performed under general anesthesia.

To guarantee even tissue ablation, prior tightening of the skin is a major factor. This can be achieved by having an assistant pull on the skin or by briefly freezing the skin with a cryogen spray. The advantage of the skin tightening effect of TLA is demonstrated in this chapter. Possible complications after dermabrasion are hyper- or hypopigmentation, exacerbation of Herpes simplex, and scarring. Therefore, preoperative herpes prophylaxis is recommended. Surgery should be performed during the winter months (less sun) and a sunscreen used consistently after the procedure in order to minimize pigmentation alterations due to sunlight. Scars may appear as a result of abrasion on the epidermis–cutis border.

20.1 Technique

Fifteen days before surgery, patients start regular facial cleaning with a gentle protective preparation. We recommend, e.g., Facial Wash by Physician's Choice (see Appendix C). In addition, they should use sunscreen in the mornings and a cream containing tretinoin or a-hydroxy acids in the afternoon.

Two days before surgery, peroral herpes prophylaxis is started with acyclovir 200 mg 5 times daily, which is continued for 2 days after surgery. Blood tests for hepatitis and HIV 1 and 2 are requested.

The patient is asked to come 1 h before surgery in order to be prepared for the procedure. This includes thorough facial cleaning, e.g., with Facial Wash. All makeup must be thoroughly removed.

The surgeon then uses a waterproof pen to mark the scars and skin alterations that are to be corrected by dermabrasion. After this, EMLA cream (lidocaine- and prilocaine-containing cream for superficial anesthesia of the skin) is generously spread over the areas which are to be treated. To enhance the effect of the EMLA cream, disposable surgical gloves are fixed over it with tape. The patient is then asked to put on a surgical gown.

Anxious patients are given oral benzodiazepine. Blood pressure is measured. Afterwards, the patient can lie down in a comfortable room for 30–45 min. He/she may be accompanied by a friend or family member.

During this time, the patient is given an information sheet about the post-operative follow-up and has a chance to discuss questions with the staff.

After 30–45 min the EMLA cream is uncovered and wiped off with compresses. Usually, the defects to be treated now have to be marked again. The patient is given a mirror and a pen in order to mark any spots that may have been overlooked. At this time photographs are taken. The patient is then placed on the operating table. If necessary, regional nerve blocks are performed.

Then we start with infusion of the tumescent solution in the composition recommended by Klein [4]. The solution is always mixed directly prior to the procedure in the surgical suite and is infused at room temperature. We do not consider it necessary to refrigerate the tumescent solution in order to improve the anesthesia.

The infusion can be performed with 10- or 20-ml syringes and a disposable spinal needle or with a pump system. For a full face dermabrasion, we usually need 250 ml tumescent solution. Other authors use up to 500 ml, but these amounts cause a more severe distortion of the face [3]. Even with only 250 ml one can reach a sufficient tumescent effect with tight, blanched skin. This makes the skin tight enough for dermabrasion with a diamond fraise without needing to use a cryogen spray.

The patient needs to be told beforehand that the face will be swollen for 2–3 days. The swelling and edema may migrate from the face and neck to the thorax, which can be very alarming to a patient who is unprepared for it.

In our experience, there is no need to add steroids to the tumescent solution. Oral administration of steroids is also unnecessary, since we have not seen any positive effect in terms of preventing or minimizing postoperative swelling.

After completion of the dermabrasion, the face is thoroughly cleaned with saline solution, and damp compresses are applied for 5 min. Normally, this will remove remaining debrided skin and stops bleeding. Then lubricant cream or antibiotic ointment is applied. A semipermeable dressing is applied for 2–3 days. As far as possible, the patient should follow a liquid diet during this time. In case of postoperative pain, the patient can take oral paracetamol.

After 2–3 days, the dressing is changed and the skin is treated again with antibiotic ointment. The patient is instructed to wash his/her face three times a day and apply Vaseline (petroleum jelly) or antibiotic ointment.

The next appointment is 10 days later. On this occasion the patient should be reminded of the need to avoid sun for at least 3 months and apply a sun screen of SPF 15 or higher every morning.

The final exam and postoperative photodocumentation are performed after 3 months. If any defects persist at that time, further surgery can be scheduled, but we usually prefer to wait for about 6 months before performing surgery again, since some spontaneous improvement is still possible.

20.2 Specific Advantages

First of all, briefly freezing the skin in order to fix it is no longer necessary. Dermabrasion is easier and quicker to perform on "tumesced" skin. No longer is there any need for a team of two physicians (one to wield the spray, one to perform the dermabrasion). Complications of cold such as hypopigmentation, reactive hyperpigmentation, prolonged postoperative erythema, or scars can be prevented [2].

Other advantages are analgesia and absence of bleeding.

Dermabrasion of a full face can be performed in about 15 min. However, infusion of the tumescent solution takes about 10 min, and another 10 min are required for the anesthesia to take effect.

One disadvantage which must be mentioned is the migratory swelling, which is due to the settling of the TLA solution and which may be very alarming to the patient.

In rare cases, we observed some nerve paralysis for 4–5 h, with impaired speech and swallowing. However, this never persisted for more than 5 h.

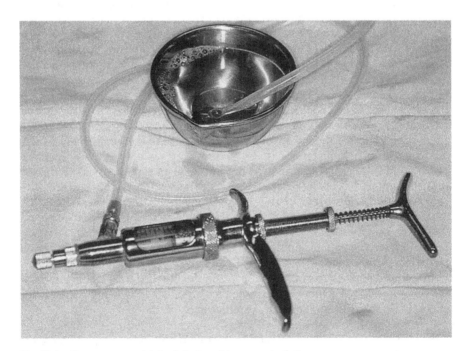

Fig. 20.1.   Percutaneous stick for infusion of tumescent solution

Thus, the advantages of TLA in dermabrasion are:
- Pretightening of skin unnecessary
- Skin freezing unnecessary
- No complications of skin refrigeration such as: hypopigmentation, reactive hyperpigmentation, prolonged postoperative edema, scars
- Second assistant unnecessary
- Long-lasting postoperative analgesia
- Good wound healing.

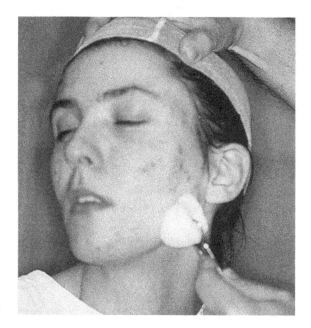

Fig. 20.2. Degreasing the face

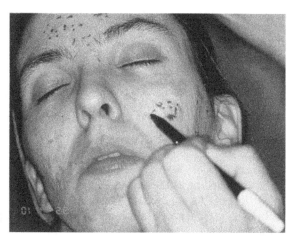

Fig. 20.3. Preoperative marking with a pen

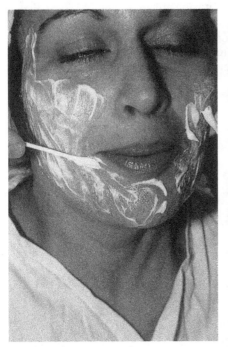

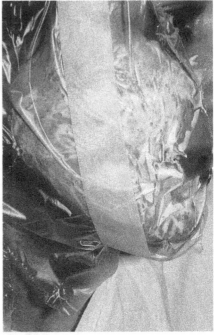

Fig. 20.4. Application of EMLA cream

Fig. 20.5. Covering with disposable gloves and tape

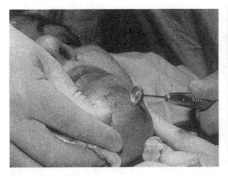

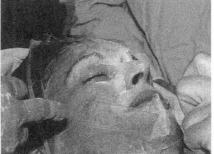

Fig. 20.6. Abrasion without freezing with crogen spray

Fig. 20.7. Application of semipermeable dressing after wiping off surface debris

Specific Disadvantages

Disadvantages of TLA in dermabrasion are:
- Severe swelling of the surgical site
- Settling of TLA solution with resulting edematous swelling of the face and neck
- In rare cases, nerve paralysis with impaired speech and swallowing for several hours.

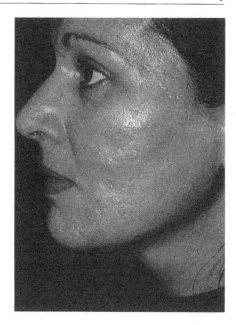

Fig. 20.8. Some slight erythema remains one month postoperatively

References

1. Coleman WP, Klein JA (1992) Use of the tumescent technique for scalp surgery, dermabrasion and soft tissue reconstruction. J Dermatol Surg Oncol 18:130–135
2. Dzubow LM (1994) Dermabrasion, taking the frost off the fraise. J Dermatol Surg Oncol 20:86
3. Goodmann G (1994) Dermabrasion using tumescent anesthesia. J Dermatol Surg Oncol 20:802–807
4. Klein JA (1987) The tumescent technique for liposuction surgery. Am J Cosm Surg 4:263–267
5. Petres J, Rompel R (1996) Methoden der oberflächlichen Gewebsabtragung. In: Petres J, Rompel R (eds) Operative Dermatologie. Springer, Berlin Heidelberg New York Tokyo, pp 37–41

21 Laser Skin Resurfacing

A. Fratila, B. Sommer

Extended ablation of actinically damaged epidermis, e.g., with an UltraPulse-5000 CO_2 laser (Coherent Co.), and also with an Er:YAG laser – so-called laser skin resurfacing – has been established in the last couple of years as an alternative treatment method to mechanical tissue ablation (high-speed dermabrasion). Both the CO_2 laser beam with a wave length of 10,600 nm and the Er:YAG laser beam with a wave length of 2,940 nm are preferentially absorbed by water-containing tissue, irrespective of the degree of vascularization or pigmentation of the epidermis. Because of this, all intraepidermal skin alterations such as hyperpigmentation, lentigines, pigmented seborrheic keratoses, actinic keratoses, and, last but not least, actinic cheilitis can be ablated accurately and completely.

Deep wrinkles, especially in solar elastosis, and some wrinkles related to facial expression, such as periorbital "crow's foot" wrinkles and wrinkles of the upper lip, respond well to laser skin resurfacing. Expression-related wrinkles in the area of the forehead and the glabella are unsuitable for this treatment, however.

The choice of CO_2 laser skin resurfacing versus Er:YAG laser skin resurfacing should depend not only on the kind of skin alteration involved, but also on its location and extent, and, especially, the patient's skin type. Patients with Fitzpatrick skin type I–II and Glogau skin type III–IV are ideal candidates for CO_2 laser skin resurfacing. From the medical point of view, large-scale ablation of ultraviolet light-damaged epidermis can provide both adequate treatment and an even cosmetic result.

21.1 Indications for Laser Skin Resurfacing

Medical:
Actinic keratoses
Actinic cheilitis
Hailey-Hailey disease

Cosmetic:
Skin resurfacing for skin renewal

With the UltraPulse 5000 CO_2 laser, very high laser energy is applied to an extensive area for a very short time, so that most of the energy is used up in the vaporizing process on the skin surface, and the thermal diffusion into the tissue during the skin resurfacing is reduced to a minimum. Use of very short, high-energy pulses allows accurate and char-free tissue ablation. The ablative effect can be controlled very well, and because of the coagulating effect of the CO_2 laser beam there is very little bleeding during surgery. The procedure is very painful, though, and requires good anesthesia of the treated area. Large-scale laser treatment, therefore, especially in sensitive patients, is better performed under general anesthesia.

Skin resurfacing with the Er:YAG laser is a good treatment alternative for patients of all skin types, especially Fitzpatrick skin type III and IV, but also Glogau skin type II. If a scanner is used, the ablation can be performed with almost no heat accumulation in the surrounding tissues. The procedure itself is relatively quick. Unfortunately, there is more bleeding when a certain depth is reached and the vessels of the papillary dermis are opened, which makes further treatment a little more difficult.

TLA is a bonus for the surgically active dermatologist wishing to avoid the general anesthesia involved in extensive skin resurfacing with the UltraPulse 5000 CO_2 laser and reduce the troublesome bleeding in skin resurfacing with the Er:YAG laser – especially if it is impossible to carry out general anesthesia in the skin treatment facility itself.

21.2 Technique

When infusing the tumescent solution in the facial area, some special features must be borne in mind:

For sufficient analgesia, the concentration of the TLA solution must be higher than for, e.g., a liposuction; i.e., it is higher than 0.05%. For painfree surgery, the local anesthetic is diluted to only about 0.2%–0.5%. Of course, one must make sure that the maximum dose of 35 mg/kg body weight described by Klein is not exceeded. In a slim female patient who weighs about 60 kg, this means a total volume of about 500 ml 0.4% lidocaine solution can be given without increased risk. Five hundred milliliters are more than enough to induce tumescence in the whole facial area.

Thus, there are enough safety reserves regarding the amount of local anesthetic used, because there is a lot less space for tumescent solution in the face than in the abdomen or the legs. Therefore, in sensitive patients additional regional blocks can be applied before infusion of the actual TLA, to make the infusion more comfortable.

The TLA solution is now infused into the subcutaneous fatty tissue with 21-gauge disposable cannulas (0.80 × 40 mm). The infusion rate should be kept as low as possible in order to avoid pain due to the expansion of the infiltration itself.

A bulging tumescent tissue turgor is desired. This is achieved much quicker in the face than in other body regions, so infusion of TLA in the face should be performed with special care. Overinfiltration must be avoided in the area of the lips. The TLA solution should be left to soak in for 15–25 min after infusion.

Now, laser skin resurfacing can be performed in the tumescent area in a way analogous to ablation under general anesthesia.

21.3 Specific Advantages

TLA is infused into the subcutaneous space and expands it. This alone confers particular advantages in connection with laser dermablation:

The epidermis is lifted automatically by the infiltration, and the distance between the epidermis and the deep blood vessel plexus is increased. By this means the plexus is largely protected during the procedure.

The reepithelialization of the skin surface after vaporization of the epidermis starts at the hair follicles and the sebaceous glands, as has been shown by experience in the ablation of rhinophymas or in the treatment of vitiligo. Our histologic studies show that the CO_2 beam also vaporizes the epidermis in the follicular ostia. Here also, reepithelialization has to start in the follicles, and the more undamaged follicular epithelium present, the faster reepithelialization will be. The tumescent solution is usually at room temperature and is a little cooler than the surrounding tissue. This may lead to generalized heat convection with a rise in the temperature of the epidermis, which protects the surrounding tissue. In addition, the deep parts of the follicles are in the subcutaneous fatty tissue and those in the tumescent area are completely surrounded by the cooler tumescent solution. This is also a good explanation why erythema is of shorter duration in procedures under TLA than in normal dermablations under general anesthesia.

In TLA, tumescent solution flows around long stretches of nerve, leading to longer duration of the anesthesia (see Chap. 4). Because of the long-lasting effect of TLA, there is almost no postoperative pain, and recovery is significantly faster.

Advantages of TLA in laser skin dermablation and laser skin resurfacing are:
- Protection of the blood vessel plexus by heat convection
- Protection of the hair follicles and sebaceous glands, leading to faster reepithelialization
- Shorter duration of postoperative erythema
- Less bleeding in laser skin resurfacing with the Er:YAG laser
- Long-lasting analgesia and therefore less postoperative pain
- Postoperative complications like hypertrophic or keloid scars, which can be related to heat damage of deeper structures, should also be significantly less frequent even in "overtreated" areas (this hypothesis still needs long-term study)

References

1. Alster TS, West TB (1996) Resurfacing of atrophic facial acne scars with a high-energy, pulsed carbon dioxide laser. Dermatol Surg 22:151
2. Bernstein LJ, Kauvar ANB, Grossmann MC, Geronemus RG (1997) The short- and long-term side effects of carbon dioxide laser resurfacing. Dermatol Surg 23:519–525
3. Fitzpatrick RE (1997) Laser ablation. J Geriatr Dermatol 5:149–154
4. Fitzpatrick RE, Goldman MP (1994) CO_2 laser surgery. In: Goldman MP, Fitzpatrick RE (eds) Cutaneous laser surgery. The art and science of selective photothermolysis. Mosby, St Louis, pp 198–258
5. Fratila A, Uerlich M (1996) Chemical peeling, Chemabrasion and Laser-Vaporisation in der Behandlung aktinisch geschädigter Haut. Fortschritte der operativen und onkologischen Dermatologie, vol 11, pp 55–59

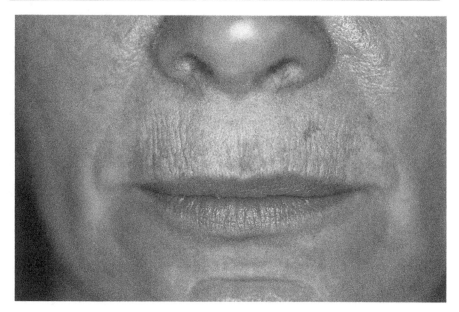

Fig. 21.1. A 60-year-old patient with Fitzpatrick type II and Glogau type III skin with distinct perioral wrinkles and a suspected sclerosing basal cell carcinoma on the upper left lip

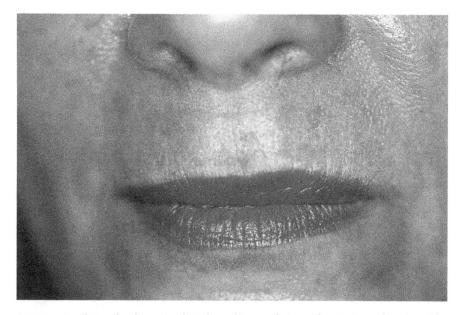

Fig. 21.2. Result 3 weeks after perioral CO_2 laser skin resurfacing under TLA in combination with dermabrasion and Er:YAG laser skin resurfacing on the upper lip. Note the lack of erythema and the natural transition to the untreated skin on the cheek

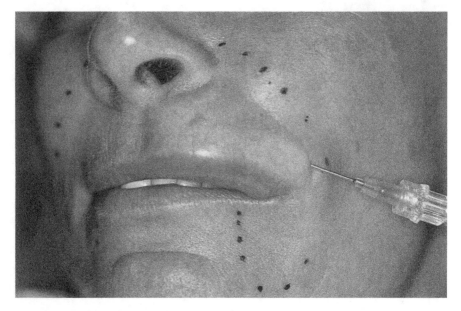

Fig. 21.3. The TLA solution is infused using a disposable 21-gauge cannula

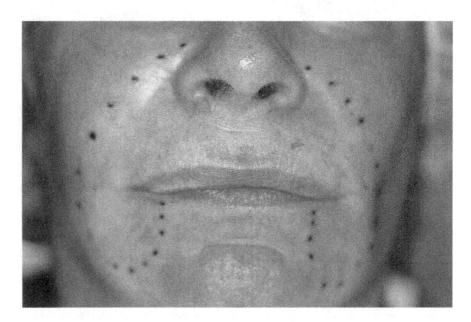

Fig. 21.4. Appearance after TLA showing the blanching effect

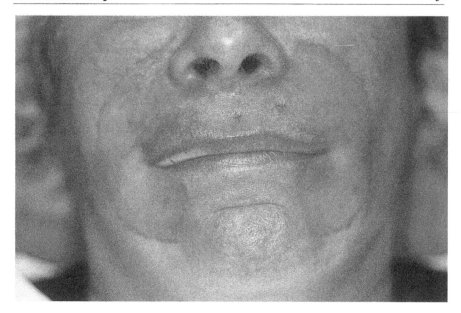

Fig. 21.5. Appearance after CO_2 laser skin resurfacing in combination with dermabrasion on the upper right lip and Er:YAG laser skin resurfacing on the upper left lip. Two tissue samples were taken from basal cell carcinomas in the upper lip

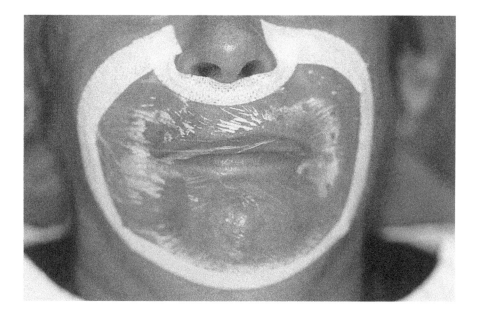

Fig. 21.6. Postoperative semiocclusive Silon-TSR dressing

6. Geronemus RG (1995) Laser Surgery 1995. Dermatol Surg 21:399–403
7. Hruza GJ (1995) Skin resurfacing with lasers. Fitzpatrick's J Clin Dermatol 3:38–41
8. Kauvar ANB, Waldorf HA, Geronemus RG (1996) A histopathological comparison of "char-free" carbon dioxide lasers. Dermatol Surg 22:343–348
9. Reid R (1991) Physical and surgical principles governing carbon dioxide laser surgery on the skin. Dermatol Clin 9:297–316
10. Russel Ries W, Clymer MA, Reinisch L (1996) Laser safety features of eye shields. Laser Surg Med 18:309–315
11. Trelles MA, Trelles K, Cisneros JL, Trelles O (1996) Soins après un resurfacing au laser. J Med Esth Chir Dermatol XXIII:99–103
12. Waldorf HA, Kauvar ANB, Geronemus RG (1995) Skin resurfacing of fine to deep rhytides using a char-free carbon dioxide laser in 47 patients. Dermatol Surg 21:940–946
13. Weinstein C, Alster TS (1996) Skin resurfacing with high energy, pulsed carbon dioxide lasers. In: Alster TS, Apfelberg DB (eds) Cosmetic laser surgery. Wiley-Liss, Inc., pp 34–49

22 Axillary Hyperhidrosis

E. Hasche

Patients with excessive axillary sweating often suffer inordinately. Conservative therapy usually does not bring them sufficient long-term relief, so a surgical procedure is recommended as a promising alternative therapy. This requires complete removal, or as complete as possible, of the sweat glands involved.

In addition to numerous published excision procedures and the already established method of subcutaneous curettage using a sharp spoon, there is the possibility of subcutaneous sweat gland suction curettage under TLA or a combination of the two procedures.

For subcutaneous sweat gland curettage, in addition to TLA, special suction cannulas are needed, like those used for liposuction. After TLA, the axillary sweat glands are suctioned via mini-incisions after blunt subcutaneous mobilization with the cannula.

22.1 Technique

Before surgery, the skin areas, usually elliptic, are marked in both axillae. For this, one should perform Minor's test, in which the sweat-excreting areas turn bluish-black after swabbing with iodine solution and sprinkling with wheat starch. The sweat areas usually match the areas of axillary hair, which are still clearly visible after shaving.

The arms are extended or held behind the head during surgery. After skin disinfection, wheals of 1% prilocaine (Xylonest) injection solution are injected proximal, distal, and apical to the marked area. Starting at these points, the TLA is slowly infused subcutaneously with an infiltration syringe (see Appendix C). Disposable 24-gauge cannulas (0.55 × 25 mm) should be used. The tumescence must be extended to about 2 cm outside the margin of the marked area in order to allow painfree suction. Infusion is sufficient when the area has reached bulging elasticity and is blanched due to the epinephrine effect.

After waiting for about 10–20 min, a two-hole standard Klein suction cannula (2.7 × 25 mm) is inserted via 3- to 6-mm-wide incisions proximally, distally, and apically. First the deeper subcutaneous sweat glands are mobilized in a fan-shaped manner with the cannula, then the superficial glands just under the surface of the skin are loosened from the dermis with a scraping technique. In addition, one may carefully scrape along the dermis–subcutis border with a small curette in order to remove as many eccrine sweat gland structures as possible. During the suction, the free hand stabilizes the covering skin and controls the depth of insertion of the suction cannula.

The incisions are closed postoperatively with, e.g., suture-strip. Insertion of a suction drainage is not necessary. We also do without skin sutures. We use gauze compresses and cellulose drawsheets as dressing. Perioperative antibiotic prophylaxis is given. The patient is completely mobilized after surgery, although advised to avoid extreme movements of the arms. The patient may take a shower on the day after surgery.

22.2   Specific Advantages

Extensive sweat gland areas can be easily anesthetized locally; general anesthesia is not necessary, and therefore the risks of general anesthesia are avoided. Analgesia lasts longer postoperatively than it does with normal local anesthesia, so the patient can be mobilized quickly. The risk of bleeding is very low because of the effect of the epinephrine and the blood vessel compression. The formation of hematomas is reduced because of the diluting effect of the TLA and the intraoperative suction. Blunt mobilization causes less trauma to the tissue than excision procedures, and the removal of the sweat glands does not result in noticeable scars. The incision scars are only 3–5 mm long. Deep axillary structures are thus spared. Because the procedure is minimally invasive, the risk of postoperative complications is immensely reduced. Early mobilization of the patient is possible, and the recovery period is usually short.

Thus, the advantages of TLA in subcutaneous sweat gland suction curettage are:
- Minimally invasive procedure
- Almost invisible scars
- Very little trauma because of blunt mobilization and sparing of the deeper layers
- Even very extensive areas can be easily anesthetized

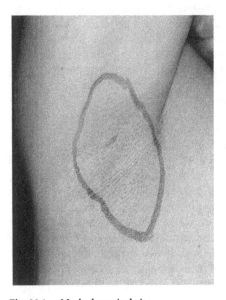

Fig. 22.1.   Marked surgical site

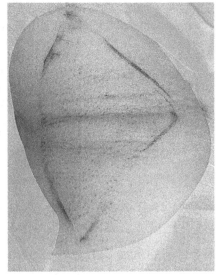

Fig. 22.2.   Marked site with tumescence

- Prolonged analgesia leads to better postoperative mobilization
- Very low risk of bleeding; practically no hematomas.

22.3   Specific Disadvantages

The disadvantages of TLA in subcutaneous sweat gland suction curettage are:
- Leaking of the remaining TLA solution means that the bandages are wet for about 1 day.
- Success of surgery is not always guaranteed because of functional sweat gland structures left behind.
- Therefore, secondary surgery is necessary in a low percentage of cases.

Evaluation of Indication: Very suitable for TLA.
Recommended TLA Concentration: 0.1%–0.05%.

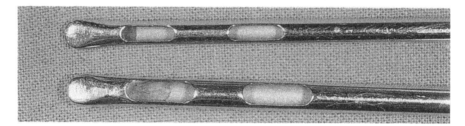

Fig. 22.3.   Klein suction cannulas

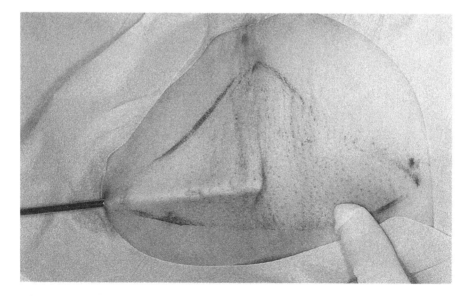

Fig. 22.4.   Inserted suction cannula and fan-shaped suction under palpatory control

References

1. Hartmann M, Petres J (1978) Therapie der Hyperhidrosis axillaris. Hautarzt 29:82–85
2. Hasche E, Hagedorn M, Sattler G (1997) Die subkutane Schweissdrüsenkürettage in Tumes-zenzlokalanästhesie bei Hyperhidrosis axillaris. Hautarzt 48:817–819
3. Lillis PJ, Coleman WP (1990) Liposuction for treatment of axillary hyperhidrosis. Dermatol Clin 8:479–482
4. Petres J, Rompel R (1996) Operationen bei Hyperhidrosis axillaris. In: Operative Dermatologie, Lehrbuch und Atlas. Springer, Berlin Heidelberg New York Tokyo, pp 402–405
5. Rompel R, Peros I, Petres J (1994) Langzeitergebnisse nach subkutaner Schweissdrüsen-kürettage bei Hyperhidrosis axillaris. Zentralblatt Haut Geschlechtser 164:169
6. Shenaq SM, Spira M (1988) Treatment of bilateral axillary hyperhidrosis by suction-assisted lipolysis technique. Ann Plast Surg 21:99
7. Skoog T, Thyresson N (1962) Hyperhidrosis of the axillae. Acta Chir Scand 124:531

23   Acne Inversa

M. HAGEDORN

Acne inversa is a chronic recurring inflammation characterized by abscesses, fistulas, and scars, which mostly affects the intertriginous areas (axillary, submammary, inguinal, perianal, perineal, genitocrural, and medial aspects of the thighs). In contrast to acne vulgaris, this is a disease of the terminal hair follicles with secondary involvement of the apocrine sweat glands. In the interests of standardization, former names such as "acnetriade" and "acnetedrade" as well as "hidradenitis suppurativa-like inflammations" should no longer be used. The most common age of onset is the 2nd–4th decades of life; the gender distribution is roughly equal. The causal pathogenesis is largely unknown; induction by androgens, as in acne vulgaris, is assumed. The formal pathogenesis corresponds to that of acne vulgaris, with follicular hyperkeratosis in the form of a retention hyperkeratosis. In contrast to acne vulgaris, *Propioni* bacteria are only involved in 12% of the cases, according to our studies; more often there is colonization by *Staphylococcus albus* and *S. aureus* as well as intestinal microorganisms. The pathogenetic classification of pilonidal sinus is different to that of acne vulgaris, but there are similarities regarding treatment.

A very important role in the pathogenesis is played by, first, granulomatous inflammatory reactions with foreign body reactions and, second, fistulas with sometimes labyrinthine branches caused by excessive epithelialization. There are different answers in the literature to whether or not the muscle fascia may be penetrated. Our experiences speak against it.

Pathogenetic-anatomically, signs of folliculitis and perifolliculitis may be found in acute stages, while in later stages there may be partly purulent, partly fibrotic inflammations with epithelial islands which infiltrate the whole dermis and reach into the subcutaneous fatty tissue.

Risk factors for developing acne inversa are obesity, acne vulgaris, and nicotine abuse.

Preferential sites for acne inversa are, in descending order, axillary, inguinal, perigenital, and perianal; men are more prone to axillary abscesses, while women tend to develop them in the inguinal region.

Characteristic symptoms are pain due to florid abscesses and a purulent fetid smell with soiling of the clothes. Patients also complain increasingly about itching, and scar tissue may result in restriction of movement.

The treatment of choice is excision of the diseased areas; according to our own studies, usually an average of 7.2 years passes before appropriate therapy is given. The safety margin should be 1–3 cm. The diseased areas must be completely removed down to the fascia. Regarding recurrence, healing by secondary intention has proven superior to all other methods of closure [1].

Acne inversa can be treated under general anesthesia as well as under local-anesthetia. However, in our experience TLA is the most suitable form of anesthesia. If general anesthesia is necessary for other reasons, TLA should still be infiltrated, for reasons explained below. In extensive involvement of axillary and inguinal regions, it has proved best to start in one location (bilaterally if necessary) and then operate on the other location 1–2 weeks later [2].

23.1 Technique

Surgical Planning and Infusion

The extent of the area to be excised is determined by the clinical findings during the planning of surgery; sometimes, scar tissue can only be discovered by palpation. Depending on the location, the patient is either positioned in the Steinschnitt position (for inguinal, perianal, and perigenital areas and the medial aspects of the thighs) or with extended arms (axillary, submammary areas). Starting from the safety margin, several wheals of local anesthetic are infiltrated with a fine needle ("microlance") in a circle around the area to be operated on. Via these anesthetized spots the area is infused fan-wise with a 7-cm-long 20-gauge needle (see also Chap. 9) with the tip of the needle directed at the deep subcutaneous fat. The injection must be continued until the whole area to be excised is swollen, white, and seems to bulge tightly. Direct infiltration of the inflamed tissue can be avoided by this perifocal ("ring block") anesthesia – and in chronic stages is usually impossible anyway because of the marked fibrosis. This procedure loosens the fat, which can then be bluntly separated from the fascia during surgery. Usually, pus is expressed from the fistulas by the pressure from below.

About 20 min after the infusion, the area is ready to be excised, preferably using blunt mobilization down to the deep layers. Scar tissue that was not discovered by palpation during the surgical planning can now be followed better to the sides. Meticulous hemostasis is mandatory because the epinephrine additive in the tumescent solution causes constriction of the blood vessels. Ligation with catgut or hemostasis using bipolar coagulation forceps have proven to be effective.

Dressing and Postoperative Course

The wound should heal by second intention because recurrence is then less likely in the scarred area; in this case, no terminal hair follicles are left. As a first dressing, one uses Betadine ointment, cotton balls, and compresses; the dressing can be held in place with gauze. This dressing technique is kept up for the first 3–5 days, after which we start using granulation-stimulating substances. We have had good experiences with 0.1% zinc chloride solution, with which the bottom of the wound is kept constantly moist via a "pipeline" (Venofix R, butterfly, 0.8 × 20 mm). In cases of excessive granulation, one can use appropriate ointment. This ointment treatment is kept up until wound healing is complete, which may take several weeks depending on the size of the defect. In some cases, the wound defect can be covered with mesh graft after good basic wound granulation has taken place.

Physical therapy, which should be started directly after surgery, is particularly important in order to counteract any movement restrictions, which in some cases may already have existed beforehand.

23.2   Specific Advantages

The advantages of TLA in acne inversa are:
- No general anesthesia is necessary, even with bilateral involvement.
- Significantly better – and mainly blunt – intraoperative mobilization is possible.
- There is less bleeding.
- Because of the reduced bleeding, there is a clearer intra-operative vision.
- Patient mobilization starts earlier.

23.3   Specific Disadvantages

The disadvantages of TLA in acne inversa are:
- Very meticulous hemostasis is necessary to prevent postoperative bleeding.
- Palpation is slightly more difficult intraoperatively because of tightly swollen skin turgor.

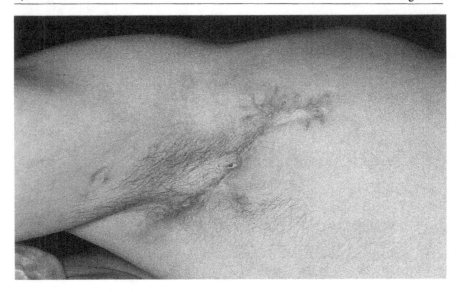

Fig. 23.1. Acne inversa, left axilla. Partly purulent, partly fibrotic, extensive and deep-reaching inflammation

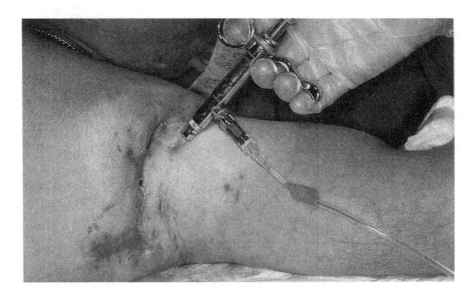

Fig. 23.2. Infiltration of tumescent solution at the periphery of the lesion

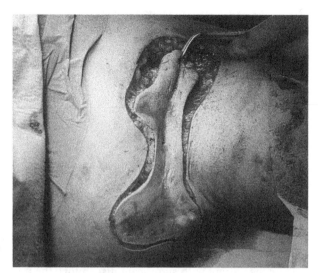

Fig. 23.3. Beginning of generous local excision

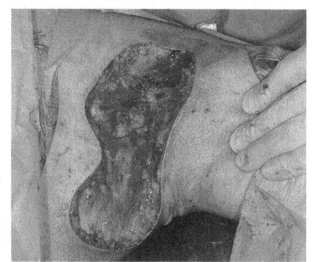

Fig. 23.4. Appearance at the end of surgery. No wound suture: as far as recurrence is concerned, wound healing by second intention is superior to all other methods of closure

References

1. Becker C (1998) Ergebnisse der operativen Therapie bei Patienten der Hautklink Darmstadt mit Acne Inversa. Inaugural Dissertation, Johann Wolfgang Goethe University, Frankfurt am Main
2. Hagedorn M, Becker C, Sattler G, Hasche E (1998) Operationsergebnisse der Acne inversa in Tumeszenzlokalanästhesie. In preparation

24   Hair Transplantation

M. Sandhofer

The importance of good, pain-free local anesthesia in cosmetic procedures on the scalp cannot be emphasized enough. There is no doubt that mastery of an effective technique is an advantage. Patients who have had to endure pain in a first transplantation often do not return for a second one.

To achieve adequate local anesthesia, supraorbital and supratrochlear nerve blocks are often performed. In addition, both donor and recipient areas are treated with multiple injections of local anesthetic. These procedures are usually tolerated by the patient with significant discomfort; the injections also have to be repeated because the effects rapidly wear off. Pre- and perioperative sedation with the associated monitoring is absolutely necessary. The rich blood supply of the scalp is often also a great hindrance to the procedure, producing a tendency to bleed, repeated washing out of the graft, and postoperative bleeding and hematomas. Hair transplantation and scalp surgery require anesthesia of extensive areas. The traditional techniques are limited by the toxicity of the local anesthetic (usually lidocaine) and the concentrated administration of vasoconstrictor.

After various authors had already pointed out the possibility of using TLA in procedures on the scalp years ago [1, 2, 8, 10], Hunstad [4] and Field [3] have recently presented the effective application of TLA in detail. Having used TLA for many years in liposuction, vascular surgery, and other dermatosurgical procedures [9], we have started to use TLA in hair transplantations as well as scalp reductions in the last couple of years; our technique is explained below.

24.1 Technique

Over a period of 3 years a number of hair transplantations and scalp reductions were carried out. TLA had already been performed for a host of other indications and was very well accepted by the patients; the peri- and postoperative analgesia and the excellent hemostasis were the main factors in this. In the beginning, TLA was combined with sedation (midazolam). In the last year we have operated with the tumescent technique only.

The instrumentation consists of a Klein pump, a manual pump with a three-way-stopcock, and, finally, blunt infiltration cannulas with several openings (see Chap. 9).

We use a 0.1%–0.25% lidocaine solution dissolved in 250 or 500 ml saline infusion bottles warmed to body temperature [5]. We add the vasoconstrictor at a concentration of 1:250,000 or 1:1,000,000; the sodium bicarbonate is also added as in the original Klein solution. The volume of tumescent solution prepared depends on the size of the infiltration area. The dose of 500 ml of this mixture was not exceeded in any of our cases – much lower than the toxic dose [7].

The patient is laid prone for a short time and the donor area is prepared and marked. A small area in the lateral part of the zone is injected with buffered 1% lidocaine solution with epinephrine (1:1,000,000) (Fig. 24.1). The TLA infiltration needle is inserted after a stab incision (11-blade) (Fig. 24.2). The solution is then infiltrated manually under high pressure. After a bulging turgor is reached, the infusion cannula is pushed step by step into the anesthetized areas. The cannula is then advanced under the galea in a second step in order also to induce tumescence step by step in the loosened connective tissue. Hemostasis takes full effect after about 7 min, marked by the blanching effect. This is followed by the extraction of the donor hair and wound closure.

Depending on the further procedure to be performed, tumescent solution is infused at two levels with a pressure pump, with the patient in pronation (for transplantation or reduction of the vertex) or in supination (for frontal and parietal grafts and reduction). Again, a small area 1 cm behind the planned

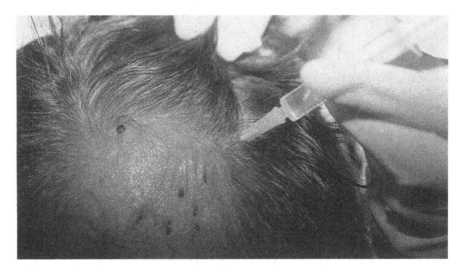

Fig. 24.1. First pointwise injection of 1% lidocaine

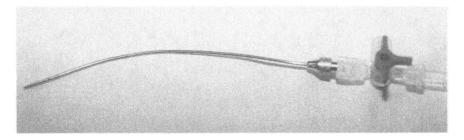

Fig. 24.2. Bent multiple-hole infiltration cannula before the high-pressure infusion

frontal hairline or centrally on the vertex is infiltrated with 1% lidocaine (e.g. Xylocaine) with vasoconstrictor (Fig. 24.1). The subcutaneous level is then punctured with a mandrin and the blunt infiltration cannula, which has several holes at the tip, and is inserted (Fig. 24.4). This is followed by high-pressure subcutaneous infusion of the complete area to be transplanted or reduced; again, the cannula is pushed forward into the infiltrated areas. Finally, subgaleal infusion is performed mechanically at high pressure. In transplantations, the infused area exceeds the surgical site by 2 cm. In reductions, the hydrodissection effect is exploited, especially between the periosteum and the galea. In addition, dissection is carried out using a blunt infusion or dissection cannula with a duck-bill tip (Fig. 24.4). After a couple of minutes, after the onset of the hemostatic effect,

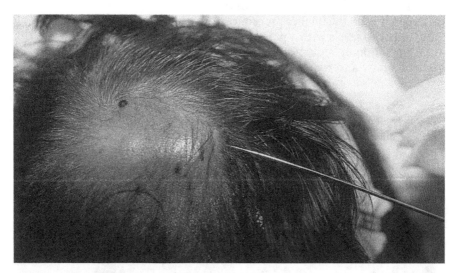

Fig. 24.3.   Mechanical infusion of TLA solution into the vertex

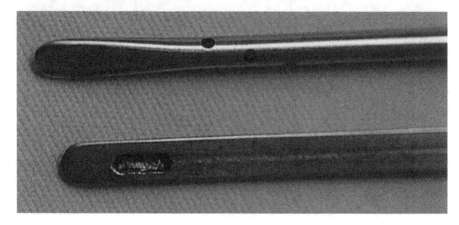

Fig. 24.4.   Duck-bill infusion and dissection cannulas for the scalp reduction (Byron Co., USA)

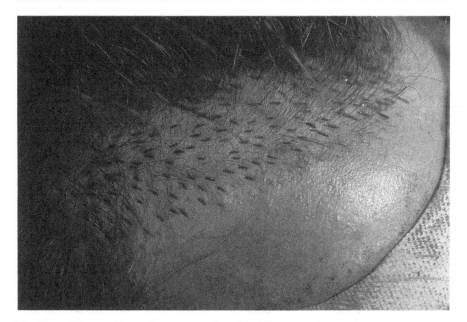

Fig. 24.5. Slots and slits on the tumescent frontal hairline

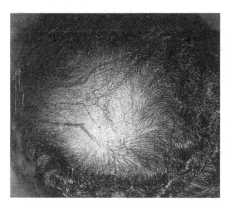

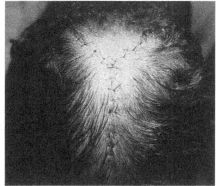

Fig. 24.6. Planned scalp reduction

Fig. 24.7. Appearance after scalp reduction under TLA

observed as blanching, the slits and slots can be placed ideally in the recipient area (Fig. 24.5). Likewise, the reduction procedure with all its steps can be started (Figs. 24.6, 24.7).

One should wait at least 45 min from the infusion of the TLA solution until the implantation of micrografts on the forehead, because the implantation procedure into the slits can be made more difficult by the increased turgor.

24.2   Specific Advantages

The main advantage of this surgical technique is the bilevel subcutaneous and subgaleal infusion technique using blunt multiple-hole infiltration cannulas under high pressure, especially in the recipient and reduction areas.

With the technique of Hunstad and Field [3, 4] complete and long-lasting anesthesia can be achieved, both in the donor and in the recipient area. After the bilevel high-pressure infusion, one has only very occasionally to repeat the TLA in so-called hot spots. Additional blocks with normal-concentration local anesthesia are not necessary.

The mode of action can be explained by the fact that the direct effect of the local anesthetic takes place at the nerve endings, while on the other hand, the massive infusion leads to a subcutaneous interaction of the tumescent solution with the neurovascular system.

The tendency to bleed is significantly reduced with TLA. Electrocaustic hemostasis is usually sufficient in the donor area; in the recipient area bleeding is quite rare. The exsanguination effect due to the high-pressure infusion of tumescent solution has proven to be not only very welcome but also time-saving in scalp reduction. Here also, use of the cauterization is minimal. One thing to be mentioned is the stretching effect due to the ballooning, which significantly improves the ease of reduction. The pumping up of the subcutaneous space lifts the dermis up several millimeters from the deep vascular plexus. In this way, surely many fewer subcutaneous thick-walled arteries are damaged during the incision of the recipient areas, whether one puts in slits, slots, or holes. In contrast to the superficial, thin walled capillaries, these deeper blood vessels rich in muscle fibers are not capable of neoangiogenesis. Thus, the elevation and the decreased damage to the thick-walled deeper blood vessels due to the tumescence helps to prevent irreversible damage to the nutrition of the recipient area.

It is very important, though, to punch the holes only a couple of minutes after infusion of the TLA, especially since the massive edema dissappears after 45 min.

To summarize, it may be said that TLA is a form of anesthesia for extensive areas which is excellent for all kinds of surgery on the hirsute head. The use itself guarantees us better vasoconstriction, longer-lasting anesthesia, and more comfort for the patient than the traditional methods.

Thus, the advantages of TLA in hair transplantation are:
- Effective and long-lasting local anesthesia; administration is not painful.
- Almost no bleeding tendency during the whole procedure.
- Due to the ballooning and lifting effect, the thick-walled arterioles in the deep subcutis are not damaged. Therefore, the punching of the recipient areas should be performed soon after tumescence is established.
- The absolute amount of local anesthetic used is small; toxicity levels are not reached.
- Sedation is generally not necessary.
- Time is saved throughout the procedure
- TLA improves the hair angle for the harvesting in the donor area. The preparation of the graft is facilitated by the ballooning of the subcutis.
- Subjectively, the patient feels significantly more comfortable perioperatively with TLA than with traditional methods.

The hydrodissection and exsanguination due to the infusion of tumescent solution under high pressure immensely facilitate scalp reduction. The use of dissection cannulas facilitates mobilization; large areas can be reduced because of the stretching resulting from the ballooning effect.

24.3 Specific Disadvantages

The disadvantages of TLA in hair transplantation are:
- Longer waiting time before anesthesia is complete.
- If surgery is started too early, the implantation procedure is made more difficult by the increased turgor in the recipient area.

References

1. Coleman WP, Klein JA (1992) Use of tumescent technique for scalp surgery, dermabrasion and soft tissue reconstruction. Dermatol Surg 18:130–135
2. Coleman WP (1993) Tumescent anesthesia for surgery of the scalp. In: Stough DB, Haber RS (eds) Hair replacement. Surgical and medical. Mosby, St Louis, pp 93–96
3. Field LM, Namias A (1997) Bilevel tumescent anesthetic infiltration for hair transplantation. Dermatol Surg 23:289–290
4. Hunstad JP (1996) The tumescent technique facilitates hair micrografting. Ann Plast Surg 20:43–48
5. Kaplan B, Moy RL (1996) Comparison of room temperature and warmed local anesthetic solution for tumescent liposuction. Dermatol Surg 22:707–709
6. Klein JA (1987) The tumescent technique for liposuction surgery. Am J Cosm Surg 4:263–267
7. Klein JA (1990) Tumescent technique for regional anesthesia permits lidocaine doses of 35 mg/kg for liposuction. Dermatol Surg 16:248–263
8. Klein JA (1997) Anesthesia for dermatologic cosmetic surgery. In: Coleman WP, Hanke CW, Alt TH, Asken S (eds) Cosmetic surgery of the skin – principles and techniques. Mosby
9. Sandhofer M (1998) Tumeszenz-Lokalanästhesie in der dermatologischen Praxis. In: Konz B (ed) 20. Jahrestagung der Vereinigung operativer Dermatologen in Muenchen. Blackwell, Oxford
10. Swinehart JM (1991) Color atlas of hair restoration surgery. Appleton Lange, Stamford, Conneticut, pp 134, 253, 258

25 Breast Surgery

R. Kuner

25.1 "Body Sculpturing": Tumescent Liposuction in Autologous Breast Reconstruction

Since it was first described by Giorgio and Arpad Fischer [5] and Yves Illouz [7], liposuction has undergone meteoric development and technical changes. It is now the most common cosmetic operation in the United States of America.

"Body sculpturing" and liposuctions, of so-called problem zones, have become standard procedures with calculable risks and results. Better understanding of the anatomy of the fatty tissue together with improvements in cannula and suction technology have led to more indications and uses. The method of liposuction under TLA, developed by J. Klein [8] in the USA and further developed and promoted by G. Sattler [12] in Germany, has shown itself to be particularly low-risk and atraumatic.

Liposuction was established as an additional method in breast reconstruction in the mid 1980s [15] and has now been integrated into several surgical techniques [10, 11, 13, 14]. For one thing, breast tissue can be better modeled after the fat aspiration and the resultant thinning out, and the nipple–areola complex can be transposed more easily and with less tension. Secondly, the aesthetic breast contour can be significantly improved by suction of excessive fat deposits between the anterior and posterior axillary line and the axillary process. In scar-sparing surgical techniques, these areas are usually outside the resection area, and are therefore likely candidates for lipocontouring.

There is only a limited indication spectrum for suction-only mammoplasty [2] in patients with a normal nipple position without significant ptosis and predominantly lipomatous mammary hyperplasia.

Other indications for suction-only mammoplasty are corrections of congenital mammary asymmetry [11] and gynecomastia [14].

In autologous breast reconstruction, liposuction under local anesthesia has an extremely important role in refinement or touch-up.

The introduction of the TRAM flap (transverse rectus abdominis myocutaneous flap, lower rectus flap plasty) has revolutionized plastic breast surgery as a method for complete autologous breast reconstruction [6]. In the early days silicon implants were the only procedure available. While today silicon implants are still in use, for this indication one can achieve better results with autologous tissue.

In contrast to breast implants, the TRAM-reconstructed breast has many important advantages: a soft consistency without tendency to become encapsulated over the course of years; it is warm and mobile, just like the contralateral breast;

and its appearance improves over time when the scars fade and the breast takes on a more and more natural ptosis and shape. Since the reconstructed breast consists almost entirely of fat, aspiration lipectomy can be employed to change the size, improve the look, and model the shape in such a way that close symmetry to the contralateral side becomes possible.

Drever [3, 4] has coined the term "torsoplasty", since TRAM flap plasty, whether as a free transplant or with a pedicle, always has two aspects: first, the lower abdominal dermofat transfer for the autologous breast reconstruction, and, second, the resulting dermolipectomy of the abdomen, the abdominal wall plasty, which often results in additional cosmetic improvement of the donor region.

25.2 Technique

TRAM reconstruction and/or torsoplasty is usually performed in two surgical steps. In the first, the rectus flap is transferred to the thorax wall with modeling of the dermofat island to a new autologous breast contour. Three to six months later, this is followed by TRAM refinement, nipple–areola complex reconstruction, as well as, if necessary, contralateral reduction mastopexy for optimization of symmetry.

The transplant flap is at first only supplied by the superior epigastric artery in the single-pedicle TRAM, or by the microvascular anostomosis of the superior epigastric artery in the free TRAM. Over the course of months, it becomes additionally vascularized by the pectoral perforating and transcutaneous vessels. Nonetheless, perfusion in the autologous reconstructed breast remains fragile, so that the possibilities for secondary modeling and contour change are limited if fat and skin necrosis are to be prevented.

Since skin sparing mastectomy is often used for cosmetic reasons in the primary reconstruction, so long as this is oncologically defensible, standard oncologic practice is to monitor the soft tissue coat of the autologous reconstructed breast by mammography, since it is fundamentally at risk for recurrence. So far as possible, therefore, any steps taken during cosmetic refinement that could interfere with the imaging monitoring should be omitted or kept to a minimum. Traumatizing liposuctions with bleeding can lead to increased fibrosis and scar formation or to fat necrosis with consequent microcalcifications [1]. Both intramammary scarring and microcalcifications or fat necrosis may lead to ambiguities in the imaging follow-up and to unnecessary additional diagnostic procedures.

Because it provides the best possible tissue protection for the transplant flap and allows atraumatic liposuction with thin blunt cannulas, we have been using the tumescent liposuction technique as described by Sattler [12] in all secondary TRAM refinement procedures requiring a shape or volume change since July 1997.

A sufficiently high tissue pressure is built up by the subcutaneous injection of the tumescent solution; the swollen fat can be suctioned with a 3 mm 24-hole cannula without significant shear forces while the subcutaneous suspension apparatus and, especially, the blood vessels of the TRAM flap are largely protected.

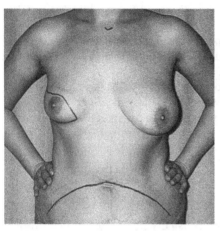

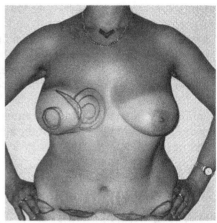

Fig. 25.1. A 38-year-old patient with extended ductal carcinoma in situ of the right breast: preoperative marking before ablation of the right breast, distinct right-side anisomastia

Fig. 25.2. Same patient 6 months after TRAM surgery, preoperative photograph before TRAM refinement with nipple–areola reconstruction (NAC) and tumescent liposuction of the breast for secondary contouring of the breast and of the abdominal donor region

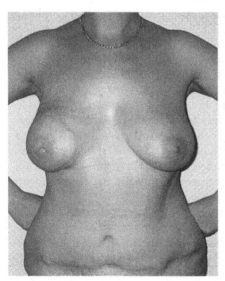

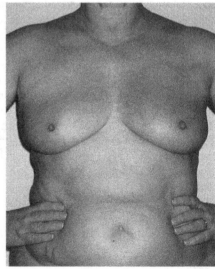

Fig. 25.3. Same patient 3 months after TRAM refinement, NAC reconstruction, and liposuction

Fig. 25.4. A 56-year-old patient with mainly truncal obesity: appearance after combined primary radiochemotherapy of locally advanced breast cancer on the left side

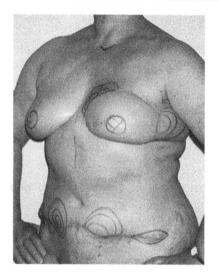 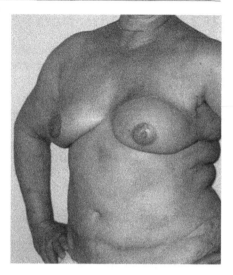

Fig. 25.5. Same patient 6 months after TRAMsurgery, preoperative photograph before refinement with NAC, and tumescent liposuction of the left breast and the abdominal donor region

Fig. 25.6. Same patient 3 months after TRAM refinement, tumescent liposuction, and NAC with tattooing

During the preoperative planning, the areas to be suctioned are marked with the patient standing upright; the procedure is usually performed under local anesthesia. The surgeon's personal experience is extremely important in the evaluation of the volume and amount of the fat to be aspirated. After the local infusion the tissue is overexpanded, making accurate intraoperative evaluation impossible. Overcorrection should be avoided.

Indications for Tumescent Liposuction in Autologous Breast Reconstruction

- Volume and size reduction
- Shape changes
  - Upper filling correction
  - Lateral "breast flow" correction
- Contour improvement
  - Lateral chest wall
  - Epigastrium
  - Axillary process
  - Donor area with dogears
- Contouring of the inframammary crease
- Contralateral liposuction reduction plasty

25.3 Specific Advantages

The advantages of tumescent liposuction in autologous breast reconstruction are:
- Atraumatic liposuction technique without bleeding or risk of fat necrosis
- Fine lipocontouring possible with 3-mm cannulas
- No danger of heat necrosis as in ultrasonic liposuction
- Technically straightforward, cheap procedure

25.4 Specific Disadvantages

The disadvantages of tumescent liposuction in autologous breast reconstruction are:
- Surgery takes longer because of the need to wait for the tumescent solution to develop its effects
- Risk of overcorrection in lipocontouring because of the surgical site is swollen; learning curve

References

1. Abboud M, Vadoud-Seyedi J, De Mey A, Lejour M (1995) Incidence of calcifications in the breast after surgical reduction and liposuction. Plast Reconstr Surg 96:620–626
2. Courtiss EH (1993) Reduction mammoplasty by suction alone. Plast Reconstr Surg 92:1276
3. Drever JM (1990) Suction lipectomy: an excellent adjutant to improve the results of breast reconstruction with RAM flaps. Aesth Plast Surg 14(4):275–279
4. Drever JM (1996) Lipocontouring in breast reconstructive surgery. Aesthetic Plast Surg 20:285–289
5. Fischer A, Fischer G (1976) First surgical treatment for molding body cellulite with three 5 mm incisions. Bull Int Acad Cosm Surg 3:35
6. Hartrampf CR, Scheflan M, Black P (1982) Breast reconstruction with a transverse abdominal island flap. Plast Reconstr Surg 69:216
7. Illouz Y (1983) Body contouring by lipolysis: a 5 year experience with over 3000 cases. Plast Reconstr Surg 72:511–524
8. Klein JA (1993) Tumescent technique for local anesthesia improves safety in large volume liposuction. Plast Reconstr Surg 92:1085–1098
9. Lejour M, Abboud M (1990) Vertical mammaplasty without inframammary scar and with breast liposuction. Perspect Plast Surg 4:67
10. Maillard GF, Scheflan M, Bussien R (1997) Ultrasonic assisted lipectomy in aesthetic breast surgery. Plast Reconstr Surg 100:238–241
11. Matarasso A, Courtiss EH (1991) Suction mammaplasty: the use of suction lipectomy to reduce large breasts. Plast Reconstr Surg 87:709–717
12. Sattler G (1998) Lokalanästhesie, Regionalanästhesie, Tumeszenzanästhesie: Techniken und Indikationen. Z Hautkr 5:316
13. Souza Pinto E de, Erazp PJ, Muniz AC, Prado Filho FS, Alves MA, Salazar GH (1996) Breast reduction: shortening scars with liposuction. Aesthetic Plast Surg 20:481–488
14. Stark GB, Grandel S, Spilker G (1992) Tissue suction of the male and female breast. Aesthetic Plast Surg 16:317–324
15. Teimourian B, Massac E Jr, Wiegering CE (1985) Reduction suction mammoplasty and suction lipectomy as an adjunct to breast surgery. Aesthetic Plast Surg 9:97–100

26 Arthroscopy

R. ERNST

In the last two decades, there has been an enormous increase in diagnostic arthroscopy and arthroscopically performed surgery. With increasingly widespread use of arthroscopy, the use of local anesthesia has also picked up. The knee joint is very suitable because of its specific anatomical build. On the basis of experience in the use of TLA in varicose vein surgery, it was logical to extend the use of this kind of local anesthesia to arthroscopy of the knee joint.

Important for both the patient and the surgeon is a comfortable, relaxed position, which may be a reclining-chair position. Before the infusion of TLA, an intravenous catheter is placed and the patient is connected to the monitor (pulse, blood pressure, ECG). The ECG monitor should be kept out of the patient's field of view.

26.1 Technique

After shaving and disinfection with, e.g., Betadine solution, first of all any existing effusion above the suprapatellar recess is punctured, to prevent dilution of the effects of the TLA solution. To do this, the patella is pushed slightly laterally and the cannula introduced into the easily palpable triangular recess thus formed. After the puncture, the same cannula is used to infuse the TLA solution (about 50–80 ml) intra-articularly. Next, the two standard paraligamentary accesses, anterolateral and anteromedial at the level of the patellar tip, receive 10–20 ml each. A 0.9×70 mm cannula is employed.

Now the wheals are injected into the skin, then the subcutis and finally the extra-articular capsular parts are incised. This is easy to feel from the changes in resistance as the cannula passes through the different tissue layers during insertion. During the waiting time of about 10–20 min, the patient should actively bend and stretch the knee several times to promote even intra-articular distribution of the TLA solution. This time is used for the positioning, repeat disinfection, and sterile covering of the surgical site.

The thigh is fixed with a leg holder at the transition from the middle to the distal third. Good cushioning is important (the best is wrapping the thigh with a foam pad 3 mm thick and 3 m long) to prevent painful pressure points. The leg part of the operating table is removed or let down on the side of the leg to be operated on, so that flexion of more than 90° is possible. The contralateral leg is positioned at a 45° angle. Both hip joints should also be in slight flexion, so that the rectus femoris muscle is not under too much tension. The lumbar region is slightly cushioned. This provides the comfortable reclining chair position.

The following repeat disinfection with Betadine solution and the sterile covering with disposable material are performed by the surgeon; the patient can help actively since the motor function of the lower extremity is unimpaired.

Arthroscopy is performed via the two standard accesses mentioned previously. Stab incisions are made anteromedial and anterolateral with a no. 11 scalpel blade. One is used to insert the arthroscope and the other is for the working instruments. The leg is held by the surgeon over his/her own pelvic crest. In this way, the relevant part of the joint can be widened in any desired degree of flexion by varus or valgus stress, without the need for additional assistance.

TLA solution is used as flush and optic medium. It is infused and drained out via the shaft of the arthroscope, so no additional access port is necessary. The intra-articular overpressure is built up by the same roll pump as is used for the infusion in liposuction or varicosis surgery.

The TLA solution guarantees sufficient analgesia for the whole duration of surgery, and continues to last for several hours postoperatively.

Because of the use of epinephrine, no tourniquet is needed, since microbleedings do not cloud the view.

Even without muscle relaxation, it has in practice proved possible to open the joint space far enough in arthroscopy under TLA. Even posterior resections are virtually always possible. A patient given appropriate guidance during the arthroscopy and preoperative information session can relax enough to allow a perfectly satisfactory inspection of the inner knee

In a few individual cases, 10 mg diazepam can be administered via the intravenous catheter if necessary.

All standard procedures such as resection of the meniscus, smoothing of cartilage, removal of free joint mice, cruciate stump smoothing, plica resection, and partial synovectomy can be done painlessly. The patient may of course follow the procedure on a monitor, if he/she wishes to do so, and this is usually helpful for patient understanding of the disease and compliance.

The completion of the surgical procedure is followed by thorough flushing with TLA solution. After the procedure, all accesses are closed with single stitches and covered with sterile single wound dressings. An elastic stocking is pulled on over the top. The patient can now get up from the operating table by him-/herself and

Table 26.1. Procedures performed under TLA so far

Total number of arthroscopic procedures performed under TLA	132
Partial medial meniscectomy	73
Partial lateral meniscectomy	14
Smoothing of cartilage	21
Free plica resections	9
Free joint mouse removal	4
Diagnostic arthroscopy	8
Resection of cruciate fibers in partial ruptures	3

get dressed. The patient is advised to keep the leg elevated at home, put ice bags on it, do light tension exercises for the femoral quadriceps muscle, and take the weight off the knee by using crutches for the first 24 h. The first follow-up and change of dressing are performed on the 2nd postoperative day. Any irritation effusion that occurs can be punctured without any problems. Sutures are removed after 1 week. Antithrombosis medication is not necessary.

Procedures successfully performed so far under TLA are outlined in Table 26.1.

26.2 Specific Advantages

The advantages of TLA in arthroscopy are:
- Good analgesia.
- None of the risks associated with general anesthesia.
- Immediate mobilization.
- No tourniquet during the surgical procedure.
- Minimized thrombosis risk.
- Procedure can be done on an outpatient basis.
- Time, costs, and staff requirements are reduced.
- Speech and visual contact between patient and surgeon throughout surgery.
  Basic requirements for arthroscopy in TLA are:

Detailed patient information.
- Good patient compliance.
- The whole operation must run to a well-adjusted routine.
- Good patient management before, during, and after the procedure.
- Sufficiently experienced surgeon.

It should be emphasized that this method is not recommended for beginners; but in the hands of an experienced surgeon, TLA offers immeasurable advantages.

27   Sentinel Node Biopsy

H. Breuninger

The benefit for patients of elective regional lymph node dissection (ELND) in skin melanoma is a matter of debate; at best certain selected subgroups of patients can profit from it. This is why ELND is not widely practiced: many patients have been unnecessarily subjected to it and its associated morbidity. After it was discovered in lymphatic flow scintigraphy studies that a relatively consistent finding was a so-called sentinel lymph node that was a highly sensitive indicator of micrometastasis, a better basis was available on which to select patients with such micrometastases. Although it is not yet possible to assess the prognostic value of this method, it can still be recommended today as it can be used for precise staging of melanoma in regard to the presence or absence of micrometastases.

Against this background, it is important to find a procedure which is as low-stress for the patient and as cheap as possible. This goal can be achieved by consistent use of subcutaneous infusion anesthesia (SIA) (see Chap. 10) or other tumescent anesthesia methods.

27.1 Technique

The local anesthetic used is 0.1% or 0.2% prilocaine solution (see Sect. 3.6). Maximum dosages must be observed. It is best to use two volumetric infusion pumps for the infusion, one to infiltrate the area of the tumor (or the site of repeat excision), and one to infiltrate the area of the sentinel node biopsy. If several sites are affected, more infusion pumps can be used, since infusion is automated in SIA and thus allows anesthesia in several places. Before starting the infusion at the site of the sentinel node biopsy, the three-dimensional position of the sentinel node should be identified using a technetium 99m collimated measuring probe (we use the C-Track System by Care Wise Co.), in order to induce the SIA exactly at the site of the node to be removed (Fig. 27.1).

First, one infiltrates a superficial depot of about 60–80 ml anesthetic solution at a flow rate of 600 ml/h (23-gauge cannula). This is followed by deep infusion of 120–200 ml with a spinal needle at a similar flow rate (Fig. 10.7). Repositioning the needle from time to time in a fan-wise fashion is helpful in deep positions in the axilla, but is not necessarily required in the groin. It is always possible to perform infusion manually at 1500 ml/h in order to shorten the procedure. As in conventional tumescent anesthesia, there is a waiting period at the end of the infusion before the procedure can be started (Fig. 27.2), although it may be shorter

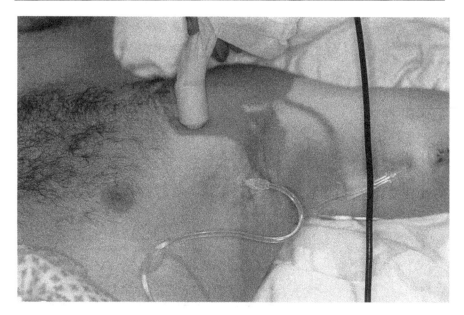

Fig. 27.1.   Locating the position of the sentinel node in three dimensions with the gamma probe in order to place the tip of the infusion needle (spinal needle) as accurately as possible

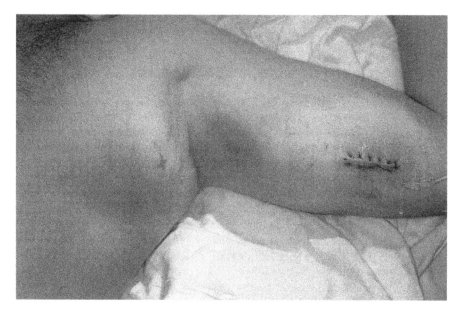

Fig. 27.2.   Parallel SIA of the axilla and the tumor area on the upper arm with two volumetric infusion pumps simultaneously

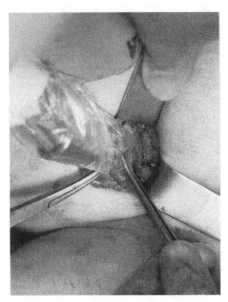

Fig. 27.3. Removal of the sentinel node with the aid of patent blue and the gamma probe

(about 30 min) because of the slow rate of infusion. About 10–15 min prior to surgery, patent blue is injected intradermally into the tumor area, which is already anesthetized; this then dyes the sentinel node, which together with the gamma probe makes it easier to find (Fig. 27.3).

27.2 Specific Advantages and Disadvantages

In the period of 1 year we used SIA in 58 sentinel node biopsies. We had to reinject locally three times in the groin and seven times in the axilla, which did not cause any problems because the areas were very small. The more experience we gained, the less often this became necessary. Preoperative medication was usually 1 mg flunitrazepam (Rohypnol) given orally. Perioperative sedation with diazepam analogues was given only if the patient asked for it. In one case, it was necessary to give piritramide (Dipidolor) in addition. Overall, patient acceptance and satisfaction with sentinel node biopsy under SIA was very good, even in the last case mentioned. The procedure is low-cost and the invasiveness for the patient is low. The changes of position that are often needed in order to access tumor and sentinel lymph nodes in a variety of localizations are easy with an awake, cooperative patient, and the surgeon, no longer reliant on the anesthetist, has a free hand with surgical planning.

References

1. Bass PC et al (1992) Groin dissection in the treatment of lower-extremity melanoma. Short-term and long-term morbidity. Arch Surg 127:281–286
2. Cascinelli N, Belli F (1993) The case for minimal margins and delayed regional node dissection for high-risk cutaneous melanoma. Curr Opin Gen Surg:310–315
3. Eggermont A (1997) Is regional therapy worthwhile ? Melanoma Res 7 (Suppl 1):22
4. Karakousis CP (1996) Surgical treatment of malignant melanoma. Surg Clin North Am 76:1299–1312
5. Morton DL, Wen DR, Wong JH et al (1992) Technical details of intraoperative lymphatic mapping for early stage melanoma. Arch Surg 127:392–399
6. Reintgen D (1998) Sentinel node biopsy: the accurate staging of the patient with melanoma. Seventh World Congress of Cancers of the Skin. Rome 22–25 April 1998

28 High Ligation and Stripping of the Long Saphenous Vein

B. SOMMER, G. SATTLER

Varicosis is neither a disease of prosperity nor merely a cosmetically disturbing change, for permanent high pressure in the venous system always results in a disturbance of the entire hemodynamics. Thus, insufficiency of perforator veins can allow superficial thrombophlebitis eventually to affect the deep venous system [19].

Economically speaking, venous diseases are among the most expensive diseases in the industrialized nations [3,5]. Late sequelae such as crural ulcers are near the top of the list for length of patient hospitalizations.

The trend to minimally invasive surgery continues in varicosis surgery as elsewhere. Since the first description of surgical ligation of insufficient long saphenous vein by Trendelenburg [21], the method of exeresis [1], and ligation of the subcutaneous veins in the groin [2], continuous improvements have been developed in the therapeutic procedure. According to today's concept of therapy, selective varicosis surgery carried out on the basis of disease stage and the individual findings of each case is absolutely preferable to the radically schematic procedure [16]. The same current standard work advises that only high saphenous ligation and other strictly localized vascular surgical procedures are suitable for infiltration anesthesia. At the same time, however, there are reports of complete stripping operations performed under local anesthesia [4,12,24] in which the surgeons have not made use of the obvious advantages of the tumescent technique.

Indications for high ligation and stripping of the long saphenous vein are based on a precise preoperative diagnostic procedure: patient history, inspection, and palpation are complemented by continuous-wave Doppler ultrasonography and duplex ultrasonography [13]. In most cases, an ascending compression phlebogram is performed to show the sufficiency of the deep venous system.

28.1 Technique

Induction of TLA

In procedures carried out under TLA, precise marking of the course of the vein and the planned incision sites is more important than in surgery under general anesthesia, since anesthesia is only induced in the marked area.

Various concentrations of the local anesthetic may be used. Higher concentrations of local anesthetic shorten the waiting until surgery can begin [17], but 0.05% solution can also be used without problems. About 350–700 ml TLA solution usually suffices for anesthesia of the long saphenous vein and side branches. Since about

6000 ml TLA solution may be administered to a healthy patient weighing 70 kg without causing any problems (see Chap. 4), it is in principle possible to operate on varicosis of any extent and also on the small and long saphenous veins of both legs at the same time. The only restrictions in the surgical planning relate to the psychological stress for the patient of a long procedure and what, if anything, is anticipated in the way of either complications or intraoperative findings, i.e., veins coursing differently from what was assumed preoperatively.

The combined use of a percutaneous stick and a roll pump has proven itself, starting with manual infiltration on the medial aspect of the knee, because experience has shown that this can be painful. This is followed by infusion at the junction of the long saphenous vein; in this way, if the cannula is inadvertently positioned intravascularly, at most only 2 ml of the solution is administered within the vein. In addition, the infusion cannula is kept in constant motion in order to ensure an even infusion. With the tumescent technique, the interstitial pressure is much higher than the intravenous pressure, so the veins collapse.

It is important to introduce the TLA solution deep to the junction to enable a painless operation in this area. The course of the vein can now be infiltrated relatively quickly using the roll pump. This is intended to anesthetize the two following areas: about 3 cm ventral to the long saphenous vein in the thigh area and up to 6 cm dorsal to it, because of the expected side branches there; and, on the lower leg, up to 5 cm ventral and about 3 cm dorsal to the vein stem and the expected side branches.

Early data, unpublished so far, show that a combination of femoral block and tumescent technique is useful in some cases. This way, the advantages of the block, i.e., good anesthesia of the extremity, are combined with those of the tumescence, i.e., splinting of the vein, reduced bleeding, etc. Because of the relatively low volume of TLA solution used compared to other procedures, the plasma level of anesthetic is not significantly elevated, so that intraoperative safety is guaranteed.

Helpful Hints

- Deep infusion in the area of the junction, normal subcutaneous infusion in the course of the vein.
- Medial aspect of the knee and of the shinbone are painful, slower infusion here.
- Err on the generous side with the amount of solution infused, to prevent pain from the rupturing of side branches that could not be visualized preoperatively.
- Always consider sedation and analgesia in nervous patients.
- Application of a special compression stocking immediately postoperatively enables better early mobilization.

High Saphenous Ligation

High ligation of the long saphenous vein can be performed in two different positions, either with the patient supine and the legs lying parallel without any changes in position, or with the leg in slight abduction and outside rotation.

The 3–4 cm long skin incision is placed in the inguinal crease or 1 cm above it medial to the pulse of the femoral artery. Longer incisions may be chosen, depending on the degree of obesity. Experience has shown that, especially in the inguinal region, the cosmetic result is very good whatever the length of the incision [10].

Sharp incision of the dermis and the ridge of the scarpa's is followed by blunt preparation of the long saphenous vein, which is located with a finger. The vein is exposed caudally by following the venous bed with the palpating finger, carefully, but with sufficient force. Once the position of the retractors is changed according to the surgeon's preference, the specific characteristics of TLA become apparent: preparation is easier because of the hydrodissection effect of the TLA solution, but the surgical site has to be cleared of fluid more often and with larger swabs. The surrounding fat appears very pale and swollen (*tumescere* means "to swell"), leading to the joking reference to performing high saphenous ligation "as if on a drowned body". Once surgeon and assistant have gotten used to the wet surgical site, the preparation and exposure of anatomical structures is easier than during general anesthesia – so long as the operative site is frequently swabbed – because of the local fluid.

The long saphenous vein can then be looped with absorbable suture material about 5 cm distal to the junction with the common femoral vein. The vein can be verified by percussion on the marked segments on the thigh with simultaneous palpation of the pulse wave or by pulling on the vein itself; the course then becomes visible as a string-like tension in the skin parallel to the marking [6]. This procedure may be more difficult or even impossible under TLA, however, owing to the increased tissue turgor, especially in obese patients.

We prefer the following procedure: transection of the long saphenous vein between a distal ligature using, e.g., Ethibond 3–0 (Ethicon Co., Hamburg; see Appendix C) and a proximal Overholt clamp. This way, the distal end, marked by the suture, can slide back into the vein channel, while the proximal end is lifted by the Overholt clamp. The side branches revealed can then be ligated easily one by one with a single suture. As each side branch comes to be ligated in turn, a second Overholt clamp is placed proximal to it, in a "climbing" technique. This technique saves time and the second ligation of the side branches that is otherwise necessary; it also keeps the overview of the surgical site simple. The Overholt clamps must be carefully handled by the surgeon, since a wrong pull with this instrument has a powerful leverage.

When the junction of the long saphenous vein the common femoral vein and the hiatic arch are exposed, the venous stump is again inspected closely, since often deep in the junction very small side branches are discovered which should also be ligated. This is followed by double ligation of the long saphenous vein at the level of the junction. A transfixion ligature through the stump of the saphenous vein is intended to prevent loosening of the primary ligatures [16].

Stripping

The high ligation is followed by exeresis of the long saphenous vein if indicated. The vein is stripped only in the segment with insufficient valves [7].

TLA allows all kinds of stripping: classic stripping with a mounted stripper head, invaginated stripping, Oesch's PIN (perforation-invagination) stripping [14, 15], and also cryostripping.

In addition to invaginated stripping, we prefer PIN stripping, especially in partial exeresis of the vein. With the PIN stripper described by A. Oesch [15], preparation of the distal end of the saphenous vein can be omitted, because of the sharp, angled tip with which the skin is perforated from the vein outwards. A rigid instrument can be better seen in the bulging tumescent tissue, like the olive in classic stripping.

In cryostripping, better temperature convection is expected due to the large fluid volumes in the tissue, in which both the vein and the accompanying neural structures are flooded. This may help to prevent known side effects of cryostripping, but no studies have yet been published on this subject.

To make use of the specific advantage of early mobilization after a procedure performed under TLA, the postoperative compression bandage should fit well. A stocking manufactured especially for this purpose with a set pressure gradient from distal to proximal has proved its worth in our clinic (Struva 35, medi Bayreuth Co., see Appendix C). At the conclusion of stripping, the stocking bandage can be put on intraoperatively with the help of a sterilizable dressing aid. In addition, we use a foam pad along the stripper channel, which helps to prevent hematomas. The junction of the long saphenous vein can then be closed and the stocking pulled up to the groin. Because the upper edge of the stocking is soft, it can be positioned even over the surgical wound. The stocking stays on the operated leg for 2–3 days and offers the following advantages:

- Slippage, such as occurs with wrapped bandages, is virtually impossible.
- Because it sits securely, mobilization is better.
- The postoperative stocking can be worn until replaced by the final appropriate stocking.

28.2 Specific Advantages

Complete anesthesia of extensive areas and on both extremities. Because the TLA solution is very dilute and can safely be administered in large doses, extensive areas of the body can be anesthetized. Liposuction is a procedure which has the highest requirements for TLA solution compared to other procedures in surgical dermatology; for this, doses of 35 mg of local anesthetic per kilogram body weight were found to be a sufficiently safe maximum dose by J. Klein and ourselves [11, 18]. This means that, for a body weight of 75 kg, almost 6 l TLA solution can be used. The requirements for high ligation and complete stripping of the long saphenous vein, on the other hand, are only between about 400 and 850 ml TLA solution, depending on the patient. This amount of TLA solution may be regarded as completely harmless. The exception to this is in patients with a glucose-6-phosphate-dehydrogenase deficiency: this enzyme reduces the accumulated methemoglobin in the erythrocytes back into hemoglobin, and in subjects in whom it is deficient, high doses of prilocaine may lead to methemoglobinemia.

Less bleeding = fewer hematomas.   The high tissue pressure after the infusion and the vasoconstrictors added to the TLA solution together reduce perfusion in the area being operated upon, which in turn prevents the formation of large hematomas.

Better resorption of hematomas = less postoperative pain.   The diluting effect of the TLA prevents rapid coagulation of extravascular blood, so that developing hematomas are better resorbed. This way, small, hard hematomas can in most cases be prevented.

Protracted effect of TLA = less postoperative pain.   The slow infusion and marked lipophilia of the local anesthetic together with the added vasoconstrictors gives TLA a prolonged duration of effect [22]. Hence, postoperative pain medication is often unnecessary.

Antibacterial effect of TLA.   The local anesthetic prilocaine has a bactericidal effect in itself [23], which is further enhanced by the addition of sodium bicarbonate [20].

Antibacterial effect of the wash-out effect of TLA.   After a procedure performed under TLA, a certain amount of anesthetic solution oozes out of the stab incisions and the wounds because of the high pressure in the tissues, thus impeding the ingress of microorganisms.

Antithrombotic effect of TLA.   Like all local anesthetics of the amide type, prilocaine also has antithrombotic features [22].

Hydrodissection effect.   The infusion of large volumes of fluid into the subcutaneous fat at some pressure automatically has a "hydrodissection" effect on the tissue. Owing to the nature of the connective tissue in the perivascular space, irregular varicoses are especially well stabilized, making surgery significantly easier.

Compensation for intraoperative fluid loss.   Because fluid is resorbed from the subcutaneous space, and because blood loss is reduced, there is no need for intravenous fluid replacement.

Low complication rate.   The unusual safety of this method was demonstrated in an impressive questionnaire survey by the American Society for Dermatologic Surgery, in which data from 15,336 patients who had undergone liposuction under TLA according to the guidelines were evaluated [8]. Complications were extremely rare.

Thus, the advantages of TLA in high ligation and stripping of the long saphenous vein are:
• Complete anesthesia of extensive areas
• Less bleeding = less hematomas
• Better resorption of hematomas =l ess postoperative pain
• Protracted effect of local anesthetic = less postoperative pain
• Safe method compared to other methods of local anesthesia and intubation anesthesia
• Antibacterial effect of TLA
• Antibacterial wash-out effect of TLA
• Antithrombotic effect of TLA
• Hydrodissection, including of side branches, due to perivascular distribution of TLA
• Compensation for intraoperative fluid loss

- Lower complication rate
The advantages of TLA in comparison to intubation anesthesia are:
- Fewer preoperative diagnostic procedures are necessary.
- Even patients at increased risk for intubation anesthesia can undergo surgery.
- Anesthesiologist need only be on call.
- Great intraoperative safety.
- Fewer hematomas.
- Long-lasting analgesia.
- Patient can easily change position him-/herself intraoperatively.
- Ideal postoperative mobilization.
- Shorter hospital stay or procedure may be performed on an outpatient basis.
- Cost savings.

28.3   Specific Disadvantages

Wet surgical site. Especially in operations on the junction of the long saphenous vein, the large volume of fluid leads to a dripping wet surgical site which takes getting used to. Because of the high tissue pressure, the blood vessels seem to have smaller lumina than would be expected from the preoperative diagnostic studies [9].

Infusion is time-consuming.   The infusion of TLA solution into extensive areas takes quite a long time. Depending on the target area and the planned procedure, about 10–20 min should be allowed to achieve adequate anesthesia for high saphenous ligation and stripping in one leg. The infusion can be carried out in another room, so that the operating room is free for another patient during this time.

Not all patients are suitable.   Most procedures under TLA are carried out without additional sedation. As in all procedures performed under local anesthetic, the surgeon, assistant, and OR nurse have limited communication, so as not to worry the conscious patient. Unplanned prolongation of surgery can result in severe psychological and physical strain on the patient from having to lie in an uncomfortable position for a long time.

Managing the awake patient.   Extended surgical procedures lasting several hours require double attentiveness by the surgeon, who has to concentrate on both the surgery and the patient's subjective wellbeing. Keeping the patient calm with relaxing music at a suitable volume and a steady tempo has proven very helpful.

Risk of intravascular administration of TLA solution.   Theoretically, there is a risk that TLA solution will be given intravascularly if it is not employed correctly. This risk is actually relatively small, because the vessels are both compressed by the increased tissue pressure and subject to the vasoconstrictive effects of the added epinephrine.. If intravascular injection does occur, the maximum volume injected is only 2 ml if the percutaneous stick is used. Because it is very dilute, the amount of prilocaine contained in this is very small and the systemic toxic effect is negligible.

Not all vascular surgical procedures are possible.   If endoscopic perforator vein dissection is indicated, this is usually performed under general anesthesia,

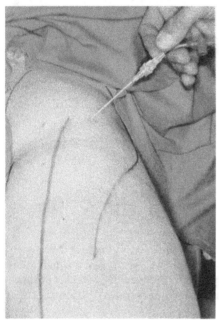

Fig. 28.1. Infiltration of the bed of the long saphenous vein with an electrical roll pump and a 20-gauge cannula

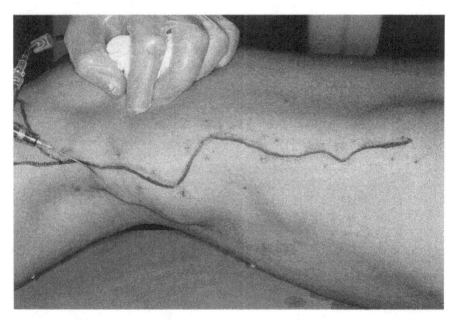

Fig. 28.2. Infiltration of more sensitive areas – in this case the medial aspect of the knee – with a 2-ml percutaneous stick (see Chap. 9)

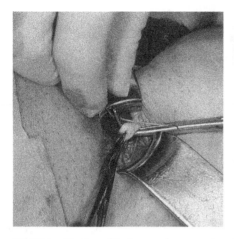

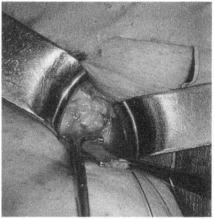

Fig. 28.3. Ligation of the long saphenous vein with a nonabsorbable suture

Fig. 28.4. Preparation of the junction of the long saphenous vein the common femoral vein using two Overholt clamps placed according to the "climbing" technique

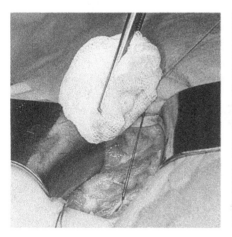

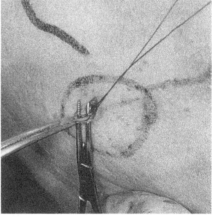

Fig. 28.5. Large swabs are necessary to absorb the tumescent solution. The pink color of the fluid absorbed by the swab shows how little and how diluted the intraoperative bleeding is

Fig. 28.6. Exeresis and ligation of side branches using mosquito hemostats

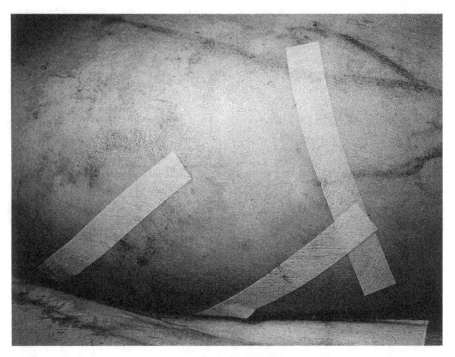

Fig. 28.7.   Closure of the exeresis stab incisions with sterile strips

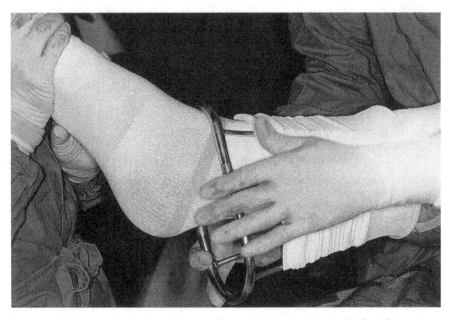

Fig. 28.8.   Intraoperative sterile application of the temporary compression thigh stocking, using a sterilizable dressing aid, even before the junction incision has been closed

in particular because of the pain caused by the application of the tourniquet. In TLA, anesthesia is only induced along the veins to be treated, which is not sufficient for the application of a tourniquet. In principle, though, endoscopic perforator vein dissection can also be carried out under TLA (see Chap. 31).

Thus, the disadvantages of TLA in high ligation and stripping of the long saphenous vein are:

- *Wet surgical site*
- *Infusion is time-consuming.*
- *Not all patients are suitable.*
- *Managing the awake patient.*
- *Risk of intravascular administration of TLA solution.*
- Not all vascular surgical procedures are possible.

References

1. Babcock WW (1907) A new operation for the extirpation of varicose veins of the leg. N Y Med J 86:153
2. Barrow DW (1948) The clinical management of varicose veins. Hoeber, New York
3. Bosanquet N, Franks P (1996) Venous disease: the new international challenge. Phlebology 11:6–9
4. Creton D (1991) Résultat des strippings saphène interne sous anesthésie locale en ambulatoire (700 cal.) Phlébologie 44:303–312
5. Dinkel R (1997) Venenerkrankungen, ein kostenintensives Krankheitsgeschehen. Phlebol 26:164–168
6. Grth W (1989) Krossektomie der Vena saphena magna – anatomische und kosmetische Gesichtspunkte. In: Breuninger H, Rassner G (eds) Operationsplanung und Erfolgskontrolle. Springer, Berlin Heidelberg New York Tokyo, pp 180–185
7. Hach W (1981) Die Erhaltung eines transplantationswürdigen Venensegmentes bei der parteillen Saphenaresektion als Operationsmethode der Stammvarikose. Phlebol Proktol 10:171–173
8. Hanke WC, Bullock BS, Bernstein G (1996) Current status of tumescent liposuction in the United States – national survey results. Dermatol Surg 22:595–598
9. Jokisch R, Sattler G, Hagedorn M (1998) Vena saphena parva-Resektion in Tumeszenzlokalanästhesie. Phlebologie 27:48–50
10. Kaufmann R, Landes e (1992) Operative Eingriffe im Rahmen der Phlebologie. In: Kaufmann R, Landes E (eds) Dermatologische Operationen, 2nd edn. Thieme, Stuttgart New York, pp 174–194
11. Klein JA (1990) Tumescent technique for regional anesthesia permits lidocaine doses of 35 mg/kg for liposuction surgery. J Dermatol Surg Oncol 16:248–263
12. Krusche PP, Lauven PM, Frings N (1995) Infiltrationsanästhesie bei Varizenstripping. Phlebol 24:24–51
13. Langer C, Fischer T, Fratila A et al. (1997) Leitlinien zur operativen Behandlung von Venenkrankheiten. Phlebol 26:66–71
14. Oesch A (1993) Pin-stripping: a novel method of atraumatic stripping. Phlebology 1993:171–173
15. Oesch A (1996) PIN-Stripping. Phlebol 25:177–182
16. Petres J, Rompel R (1996) Operative Therapie der primären Varikosis. In: Petres J, Rompel R (eds) Operative Dermatologie. Springer, Berlin Heidelberg New York Tokyo, pp 107–119
17. Sattler G, Moessler K, Hagedorn M (1995) Entwicklungen in der operativen Phlebologie. In: Tilgen W, Petzoldt D (eds) Operative und konservative Dermato-Onkolgie. Springer, Berlin Heidelberg New York Tokyo, pp 341–346
18. Sattler G, Rapprich S, Hagedorn M (1997) Tumeszenz-Lokalanästhesie. Untersuchungen zur Pharmakokinetik von Prilocain. Z Hautkr 7:522–525
19. Stritecky-Kaehler T (1994) Chirurgie der Krampfadern. Thieme, Stuttgart New York

20. Thompson KD, Welykyj S, Massa MC (1993) Antibacterial activity of lidocaine in combination with a bicarbonate buffer. J Dermatol Surg Oncol 19:216–220
21. Trendelenburg F (1891) Über die Unterbindung der Vena saphena magna bei Unterschenkel-varizen. Beitr Klin Chir 7:195
22. Tryba M (1989) Pharmakologie und Toxikologie der Lokalanästhetika – klinische Bedeutung. Offprint from: Tryba M, Zenz M (eds) Regionalanästhesie, 3rd edn. Fischer, Stuttgart New York
23. Tryba M (1993) Lokalanästhetika. In: Zenz M, Jurna I (eds) Lehrbuch der Schmerztherapie. Wissenschaftliche Verlagsgesellschaft mbH Stuttgart, pp 167–178
24. Vidal-Michel JP, Arditti J, Bourbon JH, Bonerande JJ (1990) L'anesthésie locale au cours de la phlébectomie ambulatoire selon la méthode de R. Muller. Appréciation du risque par dosage de la lidocainémie. Phlébologie 43:305–315

**High Ligation and Stripping
of the Small Saphenous Vein**

R. Jokisch

Resection of the small saphenous vein is no longer usually performed under regional or intubation anesthesia but under local anesthesia. After infusion of a 1% solution of local anesthetic, isolated high ligation of the small saphenous vein can be carried out without difficulty. High ligation of the small saphenous vein followed by resection of the stem and side branches, on the other hand, may require such large volumes of local anesthetic that severe cardiac arrhythmias are possible.

In TLA, however,, a local anesthetic diluted by a factor of 20 (e.g., prilocaine 0.05%) is infiltrated in volumes of up to 6 l [3, 4]. By this means, even extensive varicosis can undergo complete operative treatment.

29.1 Technique

Preoperatively, phlebographic and/or duplex ultrasonographic studies are performed [6]. The height of the junction is marked precisely [2], and the course of the stem of the small saphenous vein and the communicating side branches are marked with a permanent marker according to the Doppler and the palpatory findings.

After premedication with 2–5 mg diazepam i.v. and preparation of the patient in the operating room (supine position, disinfection), the TLA solution is infused into the subcutaneous fat with a special percutaneous stick (see Chap. 9). Starting at the proximal insufficiency point, the infusion is continued distally on both sides of the stem of the small saphenous vein and along the side branches. Usually, 250–500 ml TLA solution injected over a period of 10 min suffices. Because of the blanching, the anesthetized area is very visible against the normally vascularized skin (Fig. 29.1).

Now the high ligation and resection of the small saphenous vein can begin. The surgical procedure and the scope of the operation are the same as under intubation anesthesia. We often use Oesch's PIN stripper for resection by the invaginating technique. Side branch exeresis is performed microsurgically via stab incisions which do not have to be sutured.

After the final wound closure, the patient can roll over on his/her back and can walk out of the operating room unaided once the compression bandage is put on.

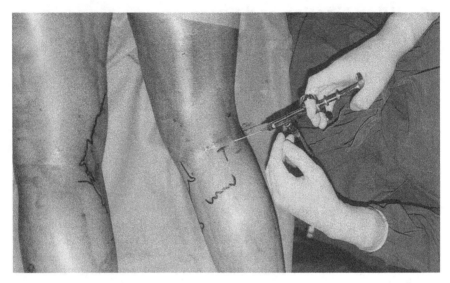

Fig. 29.1. Demarcation of the anesthetized area

29.2   Specific Advantages

The advantages of TLA in high ligation and stripping of the small saphenous vein are:

• No anesthesiologist is required.
• Anesthesia is induced on site in the operating room.
• Postoperative analgesia is long-lasting.
• Patient can actively change position him-/herself.
• Blood loss is minimal.
• Developing hematomas are redistributed.
• There are no systemic pharmacological effects.
• Trouble-free anesthesia of extensive skin areas.
• Minimal sedation is necessary.
• Patient can walk out of the operating room.
• Fewer staff are required.

Postoperative complications are minimized by the washing-out of hematomas and the anti-inflammatory effect of prilocaine [5].

High ligation and resection of the small saphenous vein under TLA is especially suitable for elderly patients with cardiopulmonary disease, who already suffer primary impairment of their mobility. Our impression was that precisely these patients had only slightly impaired mobility immediately postoperatively, and that in the longer run those operated on under TLA regained their initial mobility much faster than those whose surgery was performed under intubation anesthesia. Thus, patients with cardiopulmonary contraindications for intubation anesthesia could still undergo small saphenous vein resection under TLA without any problems.

Surgery on the small saphenous vein under TLA can be performed as an outpatient procedure. For the same duration of surgery, the operating room is occupied for less time, even allowing for the TLA infusion period, because no anesthesiologist is needed. The quality of surgery is better, and the cost savings are considerable.

29.3 Specific Disadvantages

On account of the increased tissue pressure, the thin, exsanguinated stem of the small saphenous vein is hard to identify intraoperatively. TLA solution flowing into the surgical site may disturb the surgeon. For these reasons, varicosis surgery under TLA makes high demands on the practitioner and should therefore only be performed by experienced surgeons.

The psychological stress of the operation for the patient is slightly higher under TLA than with general anesthesia, but can be reduced effectively by benzodiazepines (diazepam or midazolam).

References

1. Cohn MS et al (1995) Ambulatory phlebectomy using the tumescent technique for local anesthesia. Dermatol Surg 21:415–318
2. Engel AF et al (1991) Preoperative localisation of the saphenopopliteal junction with duplex scanning. Eur J Vasc Surg 5:507–509
3. Klein JA (1992) Tumescent technique for local anesthesia improves safety in large volume liposuction. 8th annual scientific meeting of the American Academy of Cosmetic Surgery in Los Angeles, 14 February 1992
4. Klein JA (1988) Anesthesia for liposuction in dermatologic surgery. J Dermatol Surg Oncol 14:1124–1132
5. Sattler G et al. (1997) Tumeszenz-Lokalanästhesie. Untersuchungen zur Pharmakokinetik von Prilocain. Z Hautkr 7:522–525
6. Wallois P (1988) La petite saphène: données de l'examen clinique. Phlebologie 41(4):719–721
7. Jokisch R, Sattler g, Hagedorn M (1998) Vena saphena parva-Resektion in Tumeszenz-Lokalanästhesie. Phlebol 27:48–50

30   Phlebectomy

A. Fratila

"Ambulatory phlebosurgery" was first described by the Swiss dermatologist Robert Muller [9,10] as an alternative treatment method for sclerotherapy. Under the name "minisurgical phlebectomy," surgical removal of insufficient side branches has in the last 40 years developed into a surgical technique that makes high functional and cosmetic demands on the surgeon[1, 2, 6]. Minisurgical phlebectomy allows permanent exeresis of side branch varices of both the extra- and the transfascial type, including insufficient supplying perforator veins, in one session. This can be performed as an add-on to a high ligation or stripping procedure of the stem varicosis or, if the condition of the side branches justifies it, as a separate operation at a later time [3]. Performing side branch exeresis at a different time to high ligation and stripping of the stem veins keeps the risk of thrombosis to a minimum by reducing the length of surgery and the local anesthesia. To complete the removal of extensive side branch varicoses in one session would require the procedure to be performed under general anesthesia, or else would necessitate a great volume of local anesthetic. A 1- to 2-h operation under general anesthesia that makes high cosmetic demands on the surgeon in requiring the removal of all insufficient side branches, if possible, by 1- to 2-mm-wide stab incisions, can be replaced by the low-risk TLA technique [4, 13]. Moreover, minisurgical phlebectomy has proven to be significantly more difficult, even impossible, to perform under general anesthesia. The lack of hydrodissection by the local anesthetic makes it almost impossible to excise of side branches in difficult locations such as pretibial or prepatellar or dermatosclerotic areas, because of adhesions to the connective tissue. Figure 30.1 shows a female patient in whom surgery was performed under general anesthesia and who has multiple incisions, up to 1 cm or even longer, along one of the operated side branches. The varicose side branch is still visible both clinically and on Doppler ultrasonography.

In the preoperative information session, it is explained to patients in detail that, especially in cases of increased thrombosis risk and where high ligation and stripping of the stem veins will be time-consuming, the side branches should rather be removed under TLA at a later time. If the patient still wants complete treatment of the varicosis in one session with high ligation and stripping under general anesthesia, either isotonic saline or 0.05% Klein's TLA solution is infiltrated along the vein in order to remove the side branch varices better and more easily. I prefer general anesthesia for the stripping of the great saphenous vein, largely because of the pain that results from applying the Löfquist cuff to exsanguinate the surgical site.

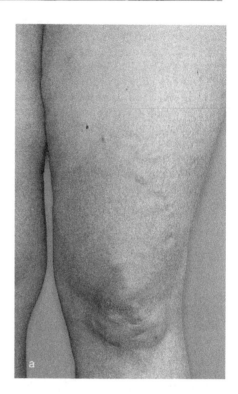

Fig. 30.1a,b. Insufficient side branch with multiple 1- to 2-cm scars running perpendicular to it. The operation was performed 2 months previously under general anesthesia without additional local infiltration (no hydrodissection). **a** Overall view, **b** close-up

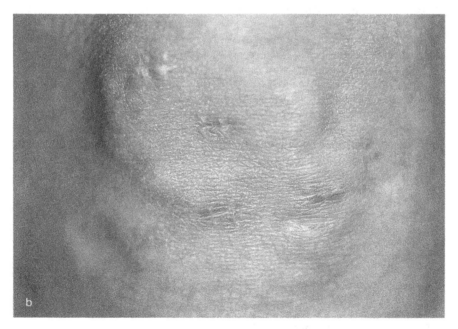

The certainty that safe, adequate anesthesia is guaranteed by using a large volume of anesthetic solution was gained in liposuction operations. This persuaded me to use this kind of anesthesia in minisurgical phlebectomy as well [4]. In the beginning, I tried to use Klein's original mixture, a 0.05% lidocaine solution [7,8], but I soon realized that this concentration, which offered sufficient analgesia for liposuction, was too low for phlebectomy, since patients were reporting pain during the surgery. The concentration was therefore gradually increased without exceeding the maximum dose of 35 mg/kg body weight recommended by Klein. In most patients, sufficient analgesia for painless surgery is reached at a concentration of 0.2%–0.4% lidocaine solution. In a slim female patient weighing about 60 kg, this that means a total volume of about 500 ml 0.4% lidocaine solution can be given without increased risk. Also, 500 ml of TLA solution is more than enough for surgery of extensive side branch varicoses on both legs.

30.1 Technique

First, insufficient side branches are marked in broken lines on the standing patient (little dots or longer dashes, depending on the size of the branches) with a black permanent marker. The patient is then re-examined lying down to see whether the position of the veins has changed significantly.

The mixture of the TLA solution that I use is shown in Table 30.1 [7, 8]. Other surgeons, e.g. Sattler, use a different TLA solution [11, 13]. The addition of epinephrine is recommended for two reasons: to reduce postoperative hematomas to a minimum, and to slow down the absorption of the lidocaine solution and thereby reduce its concentration in the blood, or distribute it over a longer period of time. On the basis of observations during liposuction procedures, it can be stated that the doubts expressed by some surgeons about the epinephrine additive (because of the danger of intra-arterial administration) are unfounded [5].

At first, we used ordinary 2-ml injection syringes to administer the anesthetic solution. Because of this system is liable to failure, I changed to the system used for liposuction, using pressure infusion cuffs. Small wheals or depots of TLA are injected with disposable 21-gauge cannulas (0.8×40 mm). The TLA solution is infused perivascularly at a rate between 25 and 50 ml/min. Small TLA depots are injected into the subcutaneous space both supravascularly (between skin and vein) and to either side of and beneath the vein. If the Doppler ultrasound study shows arteries running immediately below or parallel to the vein, they should be marked with a

Table 30.1. Composition of the TLA solution. The resulting solution contains 0.4% lidocaine

Active substance	Amount
Lidocaine	2000 mg (100 ml 2% Xylocaine)
Epinephrine	0.5 mg (0.5 ml 1:1000 Suprarenin)
NaH_2CO_3	12.5 mEq (7 ml 8.4% sodium hydrogen carbonate, Braun 20-ml vial)
NaCl	400 ml 0.9% NaCl

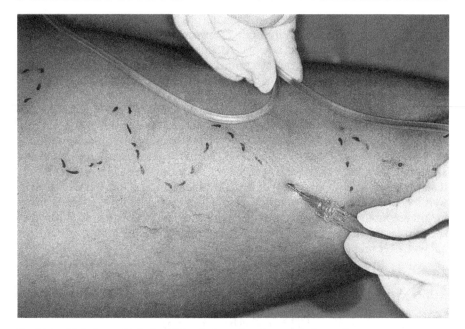

Fig. 30.2. Technique of infusing TLA solution using the transfusion cuff

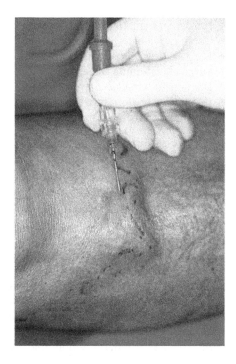

Fig. 30.3. Firm but elastic bulging skin turgor immediately after infusion of TLA solution

red pen in order to differentiate them from the black markings of the veins, and in such cases TLA solution is only infiltrated between the skin and the vein. The cannula, which is held in one hand, is kept constantly moving in order to minimize the risk of intravenous or intra-arterial administration. With the other hand, the infusion tube is compressed intermittently in order to prevent TLA solution from leaking out when the injection site is changed (Fig. 30.2).

To allow continuous painless infusion, each new infusion site should be in an already well infiltrated area. The whole anesthetized area can be made out distinctly against the surroundings because of the blanching resulting from the vasoconstrictive effect of the epinephrine (Fig.30.3). The veins usually disappear and are pushed into deeper layers by the increased tissue turgor; this sometimes makes it a little more difficult to find them with the phlebectomy hook. It is advisable to wait for 10–20 min for analgesia to become well established and for the vein to be "preprepared" in situ by perivascular diffusion of the TLA solution (hydrodissection) [2, 12]. After about 20 min the skin turgor is slightly diminished, which allows better preparation of the vein.

30.2   Specific Advantages

The specific advantages of TLA in side branch exeresis are:
- Good analgesia even in extensive side branch varicosis.
- Hydrodissection by perivascular distribution of the TLA solution facilitates surgery.
- Virtually blood-free operative site.
- Hardened hematomas and hyperpigmentation are rare.
- Cooperative patient saves time and staff resources.
- Long-lasting postoperative analgesia.
- Surgical technique easier even in difficult locations.
- Damage to nerves is extremely rare.
- Immediate postoperative mobilization.
- Low risk of thromboembolism.

Thanks to TLA, extensive varicosis with multiple insufficient side branches can be restored on both legs during the same operative session.

The hydrodissection effect of the TLA solution facilitates minisurgical phlebectomy, allowing the vein to be luxated and twisted out more easily (Fig. 30.4).

The vasoconstrictive effect of the epinephrine and the increased tissue pressure caused by the TLA enable surgery to be performed in a virtually bloodless field. The improved view and reduced intraoperative bleeding also facilitate the surgery, while at the same time significantly reducing postoperative hematomas.

Such blood as is present is diluted by the TLA solution and can be easily and completely removed with lymph drainage. Immediately postoperatively, this diluted solution, including the blood, drains out of the tiny incisions, which are left open. Postoperatively these stab incisions are best covered with suture strips which still allow the TLA solution to drain out (Fig. 30.5). Lymph drainage can be performed either with the lymphomat over the fixed compression bandage as early

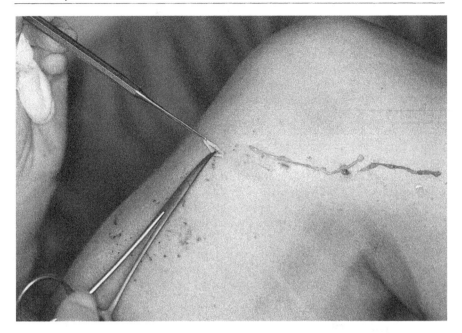

Fig. 30.4. Minisurgical phlebectomy under TLA. There is very little blood in the surgical site. TLA solution is also leaking from the 1- to 2-cm-long incisions

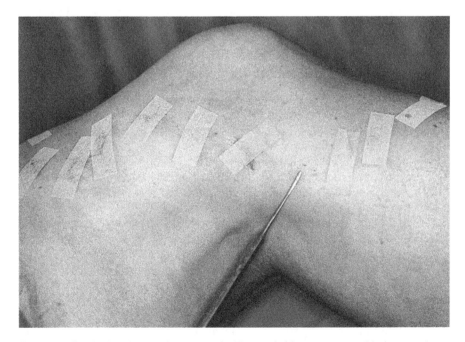

Fig. 30.5. The tiny incisions are best covered with stretchable, water-permeable suture strips

as the 2nd day postoperatively or else manually after about 4 days. The hardened hematomas or long-lasting hyperpigmentation usually seen along the course of the vein after traditional procedures are largely absent after TLA.

A patient undergoing multiple varicosis surgery all around the leg can turn over him-/herself, saving time and staff resources.

TLA provides long-lasting postoperative analgesia, so that the patients do not suffer pain postoperatively.

The hydrodissection effect of the TLA solution allows easier mobilization and extraction of varicose veins that are very strongly attached to connective tissue: on the dorsum of the foot, in the ankle region, and in pretibial and prepatellar locations. Similarly, varices that traverse a dermatosclerotic site are easier to extract because they have been preprepared.

If a nerve branch is pulled out by mistake, almost all patients feel an acute electrifying pain. This is a signal to the surgeon not to touch the luxated tissue structure with the mosquito hemostats and twist it out, but to put it back in its place.

Because the patient walks out of the operating room, immediate postoperative mobilization is guaranteed. Where operative time is short and the risk of thrombosis low, thrombosis prophylaxis need not be given.

30.3 Specific Disadvantages

The disadvantages of TLA in side branch exeresis are minor:
- Varices are pushed away and compressed.
- Early on, it is a more difficult surgical technique for inexperienced surgeons.
- Wet surgical site.
- Relatively more time-consuming than the traditional procedure.
- Caution is needed in patients with a history of heart disease.
- Risk of intravascular administration.

As already mentioned, the veins are pushed into deeper layers and simultaneously compressed by the TLA solution. This makes it more difficult for inexperienced surgeons to find the vein and perform the minisurgical phlebectomy.

The surgical site is slightly wetter than usual because of leaking TLA solution, so the operating table needs to be prepared in a similar fashion to that for liposuction. A roll of waterproof paper and additional thick, fluffy towels have proven to be as suitable as special, very absorbent, extralarge sterile compresses.

What seems at first like increased time required by the TLA infusion is compensated, first, by the reduced duration of surgery, because vein exeresis is simpler, and, second, by the fact that an experienced assistant can perform the infusion in a second operating room or in a pre-op room. If the infusion of TLA solution is started on the dorsum of the foot and takes about 20 min for the whole leg, the surgeon can start work on that foot while the assistant starts with the anesthetization of the other leg.

High-risk patients with cardiac insufficiency who are to receive large volumes of TLA solution should be supervised by an anesthesiologist with intravenous standby. It should be borne in mind that intravenous administration of additional fluid may induce pulmonary edema and is therefore not recommended in large amounts.

The risk of intravascular administration of TLA solution at any time is not merely theoretical. However, it has no negative side effects, since the position of the cannula is constantly changing, which would allow only very small amounts of TLA solution to enter the vessel. Both the arterial branch (because of the epinephrine effect) and the venous branch (because of the tumescent tissue) are strongly contracted and compressed, so that volumes administered intravascularly are very small and are transported away at minimal speed.

To summarize, TLA facilitates side branch exeresis even in difficult locations. Intraoperative bleeding and postoperative hematomas are reduced to a minimum. The danger of nerve damage is also reduced dramatically. Rapid postoperative mobilization reduces the risk of thrombosis. And patient compliance is increased extremely by the almost complete absence of postoperative pain.

References

1. Fratila A (1990) Outpatient microsurgical varicectomy. Phlebol Digest 3:1–4
2. Fratila A, Rabe E, Biltz H (1990) Stellenwert der perkutanen mikrochirurgischen Phlebextraktion nach Varady in der Varizenchirurgie. Z Hautkr 65:487–491
3. Fratila A, Rabe E, Kreysel HW (1993) Percutaneous microsurgical phlebectomy. Semin Dermatol 12:117
4. Fratila A (1998) Surgical treatment of primary varicosis. In: Ratz JL (eds) Textbook of dermatologic surgery. Lippincott-Raven, Philadelphia New York, pp 593–620
5. Hanke CW, Bullock BS, Bernstein G (1996) Status of tumescent liposuction in the United States – national survey results. Dermatol Surg 22:595–598
6. Kaufmann R, Landes E (1983) Die Phlebektomie – eine Alternative zur Varizensklerosierung? Phlebol Proktol 12:101–104
7. Klein JA (1987) The tumescent technique for liposuction surgery. Am J Cosm Surg 4:263–267
8. Klein JA (1990) The tumescent technique for regional anesthesia permits lidocaine doses of 35 mg/kg for liposuction. J Dermatol Surg Oncol 16:248–263
9. Muller R (1970) Traitment des varices par la phlébectomie ambulatoire. Méd Hygiene 932:1424–1428
10. Muller R (1978) La phlébectomie ambulatoire. Phlebol 31:273–278
11. Sattler G, Rapprich S, Hagedorn M (1997) Tumeszenz-Lokalanästhesie. Untersuchungen zur Pharmakokinetik von Prilocain. Z Hautkr 7:522–525
12. Smith SR, Goldman MP (1998) Tumescent anesthesia in ambulatory phlebectomy. Dermatol Surg 24:453–456
13. Sommer B, Sattler G (1998) Tumeszenz-Lokalanästhesie. Weiterentwicklung der Lokalanästhesie-Verfahren für die operative Dermatologie. Hautarzt 49:351–360

31 Endoscopic Dissection of Perforator Veins

G. SATTLER, B. SOMMER

Subfascial endoscopy of the perforator veins allows insufficiency of perforator veins to be diagnosed and treated in a single procedure. The procedure known as subfascial endoscopic perforator surgery (SEPS), for endoscopic dissection of insufficient perforator veins, is an addition to a varicosis therapy concept intended to stop antegrade reflux due to varicose veins. It may be performed as a stand-alone procedure or in combination with high ligation and stripping of saphenous veins.

The perforator veins relevant to the hemodynamics and hence to the treatment of varicosis are located in the lower leg along the course of the great and small saphenous veins.

31.1 Indications

- Multiple insufficient perforator veins related to stem varicosis
- Multiple insufficient perforator veins as part of a post-thrombotic syndrome
- Multiple insufficient perforator veins in association with dermatoliposclerosis or venous leg ulcer
- Single post-traumatic perforator vein

31.2 Complications

Peri- and postoperative complications occur with insufficient anesthesia in very severe cases of advanced chronic venous insufficiency with extensive dermato-lipofasciosclerosis or, e.g., in circumferential ulcers of the lower leg.

Subfascial hematomas are very rare. As long as the subfascial exploration does not extend distal to the medial malleolus, there need be no fear of damaging nerves or arteries.

31.3 Technique

An incision of about 2 cm length on the medial lower leg is sufficient for subfascial endoscopic exploration and dissection of the perforator veins. The transcutaneous access is placed about a hand's breadth distal to the cleft of the knee joint and about 2–3 fingers' breadth back from the medial tibial crest. From here, the whole medial and mediodorsal area of the lower leg can be reached with the endoscopic shaft.

In the infusion of the TLA solution, it is important to insure that the entire medial and mediodorsal aspect of the lower leg is anesthetized evenly. This will require between 400 and 1500 ml TLA solution, depending on the patient. The volume of solution used for one or even both lower legs may as a rule be regarded as toxicologically harmless (see Chaps. 4 and 5).

The infusion procedure does not differ from that for other indications (see Chap. 9). Sufficient tumescence must be achieved for the tumescent solution to diffuse well subfascially. When the desired bulging turgor has been established, a hypoxemic blue discoloration of the feet may often be noticed, but this is not dangerous and soon passes.

After waiting about 30 min after the infusion, the endoscope is inserted into the subfascial space, which is mobilized and opened further by careful pendulum movements (Fig. 31.1).

In order to achieve the best view possible, one should lift the skin above the endoscopic lens with a strong needle. Additional suctioning of the fluid in the subfascial space then allows the perforator veins to be explored, assessed, and dissected endoscopically without a tourniquet (Fig. 31.2). Because the tumescent solution is lipophilic, the anesthesia remains effective in the subfascial space even though excess solution has been suctioned out, since the local anesthetic remains bound to neural structures, connective tissue, and fat.

The perforator veins can then be dissected by electrocoagulation or metal or resorbable clips. In TLA, for preference the perforator veins should be clipped off from the deep vein stem with resorbable clips and then severed from the epifascial vein system with scissors (Figs. 31.3, 31.4). This prevents the occurrence of subfascial hematomas, although for safety's sake a Redon drainage should always

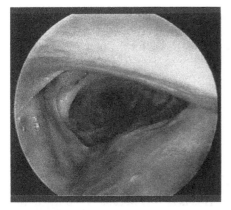 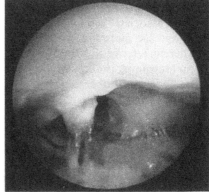

Fig. 31.1. View of the subfascial space in the medial lower leg with an as yet unmobilized perforator vein on the left side

Fig. 31.2. Perforator vein before the ligature

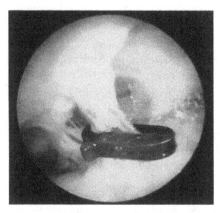

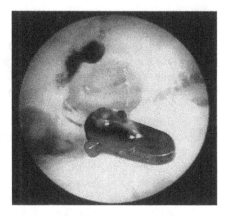

Fig. 31.3. Perforator vein after application of a resorbable clip (Ethicon; see Appendix C)

Fig. 31.4. Perforator vein after transection with scissors above the resorbable clip

be placed at the end of the surgery. Finally, a compression bandage or a specially constructed compression stocking is applied.

The patient is mobilized immediately after surgery.

31.4 Specific Advantages

In endoscopic dissection of perforator veins, most of the now familiar advantages of TLA come into operation: the preservation of mobility during surgery, ideal postoperative mobilization, and very good hemostasis achieved by adding epinephrine to the TLA solution.

Thus, the advantages of TLA in endoscopic dissection of perforator veins are:
- Risks associated with general anesthesia are avoided.
- Patient can move the treated leg and, elevate the leg for disinfection.
- Therefore, fewer staff are needed.
- No tourniquet is necessary.
- Immediate postoperative mobilization.
- Ambulatory treatment is possible.

31.5 Specific Disadvantages

Despite all the advantages of TLA, most endoscopic procedures in our clinic are still performed under general anesthesia. This is mostly because visibility in the subfascial space is better due to the patient's complete relaxation under the anesthesia. Also, there is no hard turgor of the subcutis caused by the tumescence, and there is no need to suction the constantly leaking solution. The good vascular compression in TLA means there is no need to use a tourniquet; the tourniquet used during general anesthesia, on the other hand, allows the differential therapeutic use of either clips or bipolar coagulation.

Thus, the disadvantages of TLA in endoscopic dissection of perforator veins are:
- Complete anesthesia only if TLA is infused correctly.
- Constant suction of the subfascial space is mandatory.
- Reduced view due to incomplete muscle relaxation.
- Hard turgor of the subcutis.
- Only clips can be used for dissection.

References

1. Bergan JJ, Muray J, Greason K (1996) Subfascial endoscopic perforator vein surgery: a preliminary report. Ann Vasc Surg 10: 211–219
2. Cockett F (1981) Techniques of operations on the perforating veins. Urban & Schwarzenberg, Munich Vienna Baltimore, pp 203–207
3. Conrad P (1994) Endoscopic exploration of the subfascial space of the lower leg with perforator vein interruption using laparoscopic equipment: a preliminary report. Phlebol 9:154–157
4. Fischer R (1992) Erfahrungen mit der endoskopischen Perforantensanierung. Phlebol 21:224–229
5. Fischer R, Sattler G (1994) Die Indikation zur subfaszialen Endoskopie der Cockettschen Venae perforantes. Phlebol 23:174–179
6. Fischer R, Schwann-Schreiber C, Sattler G (1997) Conclusions of a consensus conference on subfascial endoscopy of perforating veins in the medial lower leg. Vascular Surgery 32:339–347
7. Fischer R, Schwann-Schreiber C, Sattler G (1997) Ergebnisse der Konsensuskonferenz über die subfasziale Endoskopie der Vv. perforantes des medialen Unterschenkels. Phlebol 26:605
8. Gloviczky P (1996) Endoscopic perforator vein surgery: does it work? Vascular Surg 32:303–305
9. Gloviczky P (1997) Safety, feasibility, and early efficiacy of subfascial endoscopic perforator surgery: a preliminary report from the North American registry. J Vasc Surg 25:94–105
10. Iafrati MD, Welch HJ, O'Donnell TF Jr (1997) Subfascial endoscopic perforator ligation: an analysis of early clinical outcomes and cost. J Vasc Surg 25(6):995–1000
11. Ruckley CV (1984) Surgery for varicose veins. De Gruyter Berlin, New York
12. Sattler G, Moessler K, Hagdorn M (1992) Endoscopic perforating vein dissection and paratibial fasciotomy for the treatment of venous ulcers. Phlebol 23:1089–1091
13. Sparks SR, Ballard JL, Bergan JJ, Killeen JD (1997) Early benefits of subfascial endoscopic perforator surgery (SEPS) in healing venous ulcers. Ann Vasc Surg 11:367–373
14. Stuart WP, Adam DJ, Bradbury AW, Ruckely CV (1997) Subfascial endoscopic perforator surgery is associated with significantly less morbidity and shorter hospital stay than open operation (Linton's procedure). Br J Surg 84:1364–1365
15. Whitely MS, Smith JJ, Galland RB (1998) Subfascial endoscopic perforator vein surgery (SEPS): current practice among British surgeons. Ann R Coll Surg Engl 80:104–107

32 Fasciotomy

G. SATTLER

Hach's fasciotomy is one of the methods employed in crural fascia surgery and is used to open parts of the crural fascia. The aim is to achieve decompression of the superficial and deep compartments [3, 7] in order to improve the microcirculation and the transcutaneous partial oxygen pressure [2]. This will then lead to the regression of trophic disorders and may also induce the healing of ulcerations.

Today, it is preferred to combine this with endoscopic dissection of perforator veins, because the fascia can be split under direct vision in the same procedure. However, fasciotomy alone can still be useful for certain indications. Such cases will always be found in a particular patient subgroup, often with concomitant multimorbidity, for whom it is important to have access to an anesthetic procedure that does not carry the side effects of general anesthesia.

Complications of Hach's fasciotomy when performed blind are:

- *Intraoperative* [1, 4, 5]: Bleeding, damage to the vessels of the femoral and popliteal vein and artery, lesions of the peroneal, tibial, saphenous, and sural nerves, traumatization of the lymph vessels.
- *Postoperative* [5,6]: Hemorrhage and hematomas, lymphatic fistulas, lymphatic cysts, lymphedema, impaired wound healing, necrosis, infection, compartment syndrome caused by strangulating bandages, thromboembolic complications, thrombophlebitis, pathological scar formation, pigmentation disorders

32.1 Technique

See also the description of the infusion technique in Chaps. 9 and 31. Basically, the procedure for fasciotomy does not differ from that for other indications, except that by the time patients require this form of treatment, more or less extensive dermatolipofasciosclerosis is already present, which makes the infusion of TLA solution more difficult. Because of the reduced elasticity of the subcutaneous space, a very slow infusion rate should be chosen. It is important to ensure that sufficient tumescence is induced, so that the TLA solution can diffuse subfascially. In some cases it is advisable to infuse only a little tumescent solution at first, wait for about 15 min, then repeat the process once or twice more.

Once the desired bulging turgor has been induced, a hypoxemic blue discoloration of the feet often becomes noticeable; this is not dangerous and soon passes.

After waiting for the TLA to take effect, the surgical procedure can be performed as described by Hach [2], as follows:

An incision about 4 cm long is made on the medial aspect of the lower leg, and the fascia is opened and split using the special instruments developed by Hach (Martin Co., Tuttlingen, Germany). Then, the surgeon runs down the subfascial space with the dissection spatula to disrupt the perforator veins. A compression bandage is applied after surgery.

32.2 Specific Advantages

Because of the good hemostatic effect of TLA, a tourniquet is not necessary. As in all procedures under TLA, the patient can be mobilized immediately postoperatively. The further postoperative course is characterized by longer-lasting analgesia and fewer hematomas.

32.3 Specific Disadvantages

A tourniquet cannot be applied, even if it is needed in certain cases. If intraoperative complications arise in surgery under general anesthesia, the operation can be extended; in TLA, on the other hand, one can only treat the area that has already been anesthetized.

References

1. Fischer R (1992) Erfahrungen mit der endoskopischen Perforantensanierung. Phlebol 21:224–229
2. Hach W, Hach-Wunderle V (1994) Die Rezirkulationskreise der primären Varikose – pathophysiologische Grundlagen zur operativen Therapie. Springer, Berlin Heidelberg New York Tokyo, pp 61–65
3. Hach W, Vanderpuye R (1985) Operationstechnik der paratibialen Fasziotomie. Med Welt 36:1616–1618
4. Hagmüller GW (1992) Komplikationen bei der Chirurgie der Varikose. Langenbecks Arch Suppl Kongressbd 470:4
5. Helmig L, Stelzer G, Ehresmann U, Salzmann P (1983) Verletzungen der tiefen Venen bei Krampfaderoperationen. Chirurg 54:118–123
6. Horsch S (1988) Operative Fehler und Komplikationen (Venenchirurgie). Langenbecks Arch Chir, Suppl II (Kongressbericht):153–156
7. Langer C, Fischer R, Fratila A et al (1997) Leitlinien zur operativen Behandlung von Venenkrankheiten. Phlebol 26: 66–71

33   Debridement of Venous Ulcers

M. Augustin, W. Vanscheidt

Even today, the treatment of chronic wounds is still a special challenge for every therapist. The most common chronic wounds are crural (leg) ulcers, decubital ulcers, and other ulcers caused by vascular processes.

There is now an international consensus that one of the most important measures in the treatment of ulcers is early and repeated debridement. Despite many innovations in enzymatic debridement, surgical wound debridement is still the mainstay for practically all ulcerating wounds.

Since chronic ulcers often are very extensive and painful, surgical treatment under local anesthesia is often out of the question. Even the application of local anesthetic ointments (e.g., Emla cream, containing 2.5% each of lidocaine and prilocaine) does not usually suffice. Therefore, patients with wounds that need to be debrided have often had to undergo surgery under regional or general anesthesia. Because many of the patients are suffering multiple morbidities, these forms of anesthesia are often very resource-intensive and comparatively risky, especially since the debridements usually have to be repeated after a couple of days. The question therefore arose as to whether TLA could fill this gap and simplify anesthesia in surgical wound debridement.

In the literature on TLA, debridement has not yet been investigated systematically as a possible indication (as of June 1998). It was mentioned in the review article by Sommer and Sattler [1]. Many of the more recent works on debridement of chronic wounds do not yet mention this technique of anesthesia.

This chapter contains a report summarizing the experiences gained so far in treating chronic wounds under TLA at the Freiburg outpatient wound clinic and the Department of Surgical Dermatology.

32.1   Technique

The TLA solution was mixed following Sommer and Sattler [1]. 50 ml 1% prilocaine, 6 ml sodium bicarbonate, and 1 ml epinephrine 1:1000 were added to 1 l physiologic saline solution. The TLA solution was manually injected with a 20-ml infusion syringe and a three-way stopcock or with an injection syringe with a unidirectional valve. The injections were done into the subcutaneous tissue from the healthy margin of the ulcer and usually undermined the ulcer. The aim was to achieve a bulging elastic turgor of the skin and the subcutis. The volume used ranged from 200 to 800 ml on the lower leg and 500 to 1200 ml on the thigh and trunk.

After administration of the tumescent solution, we waited 40–60 min before starting surgery.

32.2 Specific Advantages

Overall, the TLA technique has proven very practical, less resource-intensive than regional or general anesthesia, and gentler on the patients.

No serious side effects occurred in our patients. The analgesia usually lasted for several hours after the procedure.

32.3 Specific Disadvantages

In cases of severe dermatoliposclerosis or circumferential ulcers, satisfactory anesthesia cannot always be achieved.

32.4 Clinical Study

Patients and Treatment

About 600 patients with chronic wounds of all kinds are treated at the Freiburg outpatient wound clinic every year. A large part of the caseload relates to the treatment of crural ulcers. All patients consecutively undergo basic documentation and, since 1996, debridement under TLA if appropriate.

During the course of this study, 26 patients underwent a total of 41 debridements. The diagnoses were as follows: venous crural ulcer ($n=9$), mixed crural ulcer ($n=4$), decubital ulcers ($n=6$), vasculitic ulcers ($n=2$), ulcers following arterial embolism of the cutaneous blood vessels ($n=3$), paraneoplastic ulcers ($n=2$).

Results

The descriptive assessment showed that for the majority of ulcerated wounds good anesthesia was attained with TLA with comparatively little stress for the patients. Thighs, calves, and trunk were better suited for the administration of TLA solution than the medial and lateral aspects of the lower leg. Infusion of the solution was especially difficult in circumferential ulcers of the lower leg or severe dermatoliposclerosis. In several such cases, complete anesthesia could not be achieved.

The success of the TLA method therefore depends less on the nature of the wound than on the nature of its surroundings and its location.

The attempt to apply a cuff-like depot of TLA solution in the healthy skin proximal to a dermatoliposclerotic crural ulcer was also unsatisfying. The effect of a complete nerve block was reproduced.

For decubital ulcers on the back, the TLA technique provided good analgesia for debridement in all cases, even where ulceration was extensive. The same was true for all other wounds so long as there was sufficient subcutaneous fat beneath them.

Among ulcers of the lower extremity with arterial involvement, some patients experienced pain – in some cases quite severe – during the waiting period after infusion of the anesthetic. This was probably due to the vasoconstriction caused by the epinephrine. However, the pain diminished in the course of the anesthesia.

Discussion

In a first open clinical trial, patients with ulcers of varying etiology were subjected to debridement under TLA. So long as a sufficient volume of TLA solution could be injected into the subcutaneous space, this technique provided good anesthetic effect which allowed the debridement to be performed without any problems. In these patients, TLA has proven to be a real alternative to regional and general anesthesia. In addition to the reduced stress for the patient, the small amount of bleeding during debridement with a scalpel, curette, or scissors was another advantage.

Since a significant percentage of patients with crural ulcers have marked dermatoliposclerotic alterations on their lower legs, however, TLA cannot be made a general recommendation for ulcer debridement. Rather, each case should be assessed individually and other techniques of anesthesia used if necessary. Where only a partial effect is achieved with TLA, the additive effect of combination with another local anesthetic, e.g., a suitable local anesthetic ointment, may be satisfactory.

To summarize, it may be said that the TLA technique is an aid in surgical wound debridement. Considering the importance of surgical debridement of chronic wounds and the fact that it often has to be performed several times in each patient, the introduction of TLA can be regarded as a qualitatively significant factor that probably also has economic relevance. In the future, one question that needs in-

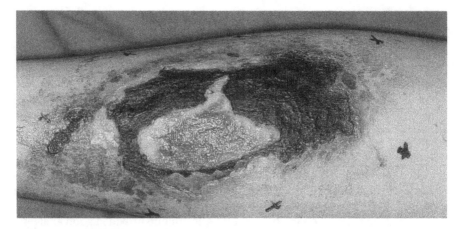

Fig. 33.1. Necrotic ulcer before debridement

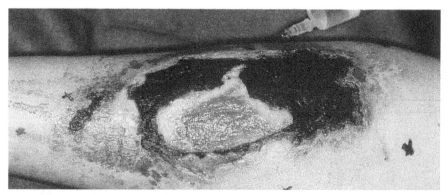

Fig. 33.2. Administration of TLA

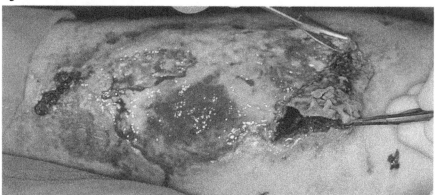

Fig. 33.3. Surgical debridement

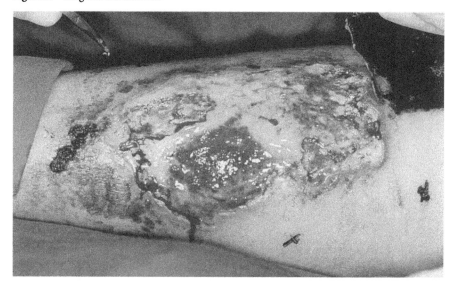

Fig. 33.4. Appearance after debridement: necrosis and coating have been largely ablated

vestigation is to what extent TLA, especially the added epinephrine, has a negative effect on wound healing. It is a possible effect, as a result of either the epinephrine or the depolarizing effect of the local anesthetic. However, no such effects have yet been observed clinically.

References

1. Sommer B, Sattler G (1998) Tumeszenzlokalanästhesie. Weiterentwicklung der Lokalanästhesieverfahren für die operative Dermatologie. Hautarzt 49: 351–360

34   Shave Therapy for Crural Ulcers

W. Schmeller

Crural ulcers associated with epifascial and transfascial venous insufficiency can usually be treated causally and effectively with standard surgical techniques [6]. Ulcers associated with subfascial venous insufficiency, on the other hand, are a great therapeutic problem. Since neither the dilation in cases of primary insufficiency of the main veins nor the irreversible damage to the deep venous system in post-thrombotic syndrome can be treated causally with surgery, compression is regarded as the therapy of choice worldwide. By this means, about 80% of all venous ulcers can be healed [11].

In surgical procedures, healing time can be reduced by covering clean granulating ulcers with split-thickness grafts [7,21]. Other established invasive measures – sometimes performed endoscopically – are paratibial fasciotomy with perforator dissection in medial ulcers [5, 6, 23] and ulcer-scar-fascia excision [9] or crural fasciotomy [6, 20].

An alternative to the last two methods that has proved its worth is extended ablation of the ulcers together with the surrounding dermatoliposclerosis without opening or removing the fascia [4]. Under the name "shave therapy", this method has become increasingly popular in recent years [18].

34.1   Shave Therapy

Indications

Shave therapy is primarily indicated in cases of refractory or chronic recurring ulcers caused by deep venous insufficiency. "Refractory" means that with the best treatment no improvement is seen within 3 months or healing is not achieved within 12 months [3]. The technique is also suitable for recurrences after paratibial fasciotomy and/or perforator dissection and for ulcers affecting the entire circumference of the lower leg.

Good results were also achieved in venous–arterial mixed ulcers –and a few isolated cases of purely arterial ulcers – in patients with peripheral arterial vascular occlusion that was either inoperable or unresponsive to conservative treatment. Whether shave therapy is also suitable for neurotrophic ulcers and for ulcers associated with livedo vasculitis [2] cannot yet be definitively stated because too few cases have been observed so far.

Contraindications

As for all surgical procedures, contraindications include acute inflammatory changes. The ulcer should not be, or be only slightly, layered or contaminated. Any bacterial (erysipelas, folliculitis) or a bacterial inflammation (contact eczema, allergic vasculitis) in the surrounding tissues should have healed.

Preparation for Surgery

Preoperatively, the ulcer is cleaned of fibrinous or necrotic layers, and a culture swab is taken from the bottom of the ulcer for microorganism identification and resistance testing. One day before surgery, povidone-iodine (Betadine ointment or solution) or a similar preparation may be applied. Complete sterility is not necessary and is probably impossible to achieve. Since postoperative wound infections are very rare (occurring in only about 2% of our patients), we do not give peri- or postoperative antibiotic prophylaxis.

Postoperative Care

After surgery, a compression bandage is wrapped around the leg up to the thigh. For patients with peripheral vascular occlusion, only a loose bandage is applied. We recommend that patients should not be allowed to get up for 2–3 days postoperatively, but they may move about in bed and do movement exercises as part of physical thrombosis prophylaxis; complete sedation of the patients – who are usually elderly – or fixation of the operated extremity or extremities is purposely avoided. The first dressing changes are on the 3rd and 5th postoperative days. As medication, we give low-dose heparin subcutaneously.

Combination with Other Surgical Procedures

If photoplethysmography or phlebodynamometry reveals improvable venous insufficiency, the insufficient epifascial or transfascial veins may be removed or ligated in addition to the shave therapy.

Possible Problems and Complications

Infra- and retromalleolar ulcers are usually slightly more difficult to ablate than supramalleolar ulcers. Although this region is smoothed out in the majority of patients with venous disease by the swelling of the lower leg, it can nevertheless be more difficult to shave the ulcer and model the wound base with the large dermatome; for this, the small manual dermatome with only a 3.5-cm-long (razor) blade can sometimes be helpful.

In the removal of sclerosis down to the deeper layers of the subcutis, sensitive nerves are severed, which can lead to disturbed sensation in the transplanted area. Our patients only mentioned these in response to detailed questioning, and consistently described them as "not disturbing". Such disturbances of sensation were recorded in 38% of patients. Similar disturbances of sensation in the lower leg were reported by patients after excision of melanomas down to the fascia followed by split-thickness graft.

If ablation with the dermatome goes too deep, the tendon of the anterior tibial muscle or the Achilles tendon may be exposed. The latter is especially possible with circumferential lower leg ulcers.

Results

From January 1994 to October 1998, at the Dermatology Department of the University of Lübeck we employed shave therapy to treat a total of 124 patients with subfascial venous insufficiency. They had a total of 162 refractory ulcers on 109 extremities. Figures 34.3–6 show the course of treatment in some of the cases.

Analysis of the short-term results showed that 3 months postoperatively the ulcers or defects were completely closed in 79% of the patients [19].

In April 1998, follow-up examinations were performed in order to assess the long-term results in the first 41 patients, treated between 1994 and 1996. Their average age was 70 years (range 52–87 years) and the average age of the ulcers was 20 years (range 0.5–65 years).

A total of 75 ulcers on 51 extremities had been treated. The average postoperative observation period was 2 years and 5 months (range 1 year and 3 months to 4 years and 3 months). The ulcers were completely closed in 67% of the patients. The healing rate was 76% in patients with primary vein stem insufficiency and 58% in patients with post-thrombotic syndrome. Some of the patients with venous disease who suffered recurrences had failed to apply compression consistently. The size of remaining or recurring ulcers was 10%–20% of the initial finding. Bearing in mind that this was a group of "problem" patients with "incurable" ulcers, the late results may be regarded as extremely good. All patients – with long histories of persistent, and in some cases enormous ulcers, and often multiple frustrated previous attempts at therapy–assessed the surgical result as "good" or "very good".

For mixed arterial–venous ulcers (Fig. 34.6) follow-up studies over up to 2.5 years exist; for purely arterial ulcers (Fig. 34.7) follow-up studies up to 1 year (for the latter only a few individual case observations exist).

Pathophysiologic Principles

Dermatosclerosis or dermatoliposclerosis in the area of the distal half of the lower leg is a pathognomonic finding in patients with stage II and III chronic venous insufficiency. Today, we know that the bone-like consistency of the sclerotic tissue is a result of the changes in the collagen cross-connections [1]. The extent and degree of this induration of the skin and subcutis increase with the severity of chronic venous insufficiency. CT and MRI studies have shown that venous ulcers only develop where there is underlying dermatoliposclerosis [15, 16, 20]. It has been demonstrated with 20-MHz ultrasonography that the sclerosis starts in the upper layers of the dermis and then spreads to the deeper layers; later, the upper and finally the deeper layers of the subcutis and the fascia (dermatolipofascio-sclerosis) are included in the sclerotic process [24]. This may only take a couple of years in cases of post-thrombotic syndrome [8].

Histological and electron microscopic studies of the indurated dermis and subcutis show glomerulus-like deformations of the blood vessels with thickening of the walls and swelling of the endothelial cells, capillary rarefaction, microthrombi and infarcts, pericapillary vascular sheaths (formed of fibrin, pericytes, and fibroblasts), and an increase in homogenized collagen fibers, often in combination with lymphohistiocytic infiltrates [10, 22, 24].

These macro- and micromorphologic features are accompanied by functional changes that manifest as an increase in the laser Doppler flux and a decrease in the cutaneous partial oxygen pressure in the area of the dermatoliposclerosis, especially around the ulcer [13, 14, 17]. Pathophysiologically, it is the trophic disorders in the sclerotic tissue that determine the development and persistence of venous ulcers [12].

These tissue structures are (largely) removed by shave therapy. In this way wound healing is shifted from a superficial area with "poor" microcirculation to a deeper area with "better" microcirculation. In studies performed preoperatively on the ulcer margin and 3 months postoperatively at the identical location on the split-thickness graft, both the laser Doppler flux and the transcutaneous and intracutaneous partial oxygen pressure showed postoperative improvement, with significant differences from the initial findings [18].

Thus, shave therapy differs fundamentally from split-thickness graft after conservative wound cleaning and granulation without removal of the surrounding sclerosis [7]. The latter method has been called "fast-forward ulcer healing", but shows poor short- and long-term results [21].

The improvement of the microcirculation must not, however, obscure the fact that the disturbed venous macrocirculation is not influenced by shave therapy. It is a purely symptomatic treatment that can – if possible – be combined with ligation or dissection of transfascial veins. In order to prevent recurrence of the dermatoliposclerosis and the ulcers, further consistent compression treatment is necessary in all cases.

34.2 Technique

The majority of patients treated in Lübeck since 1994 underwent surgery under intubation or epidural anesthesia. In the last couple of months, local anesthesia has been increasingly used, both in the conventional form and using tumescent technique according to Sattler.

In the conventional form of local anesthesia, a relatively small volume of a relatively highly concentrated solution is injected at multiple sites into the indurated area and under the ulcer. Despite an enormous effort of strength, this is often difficult to perform in the hardened tissue and is unpleasant for both the doctor and the patient.

Infusion Technique

Since in TLA a relatively large volume of low-concentration solution is available, the injection can be placed at a single site proximal to the indurated area; the whole surgical site is anesthetized by painless diffusion of the solution. The process can be accelerated by having the patient sit with legs dangling. This procedure has been used even in elderly patients for whom the anesthesiologist ruled out intubation anesthesia on the basis of cardiac or pulmonary problems.

Surgical Technique

In shave therapy, both ulcers and the surrounding dermatoliposclerosis are removed with the Schink manual dermatome (blade length 10 cm) or with an electrodermatome. If possible, the entire indurated and trophically destroyed tissue adjacent to and beneath the ulcer should be ablated horizontally from the outside to the inside in thin slices (Fig. 34.1b). The manual dermatome is set to the largest slice thickness; the actual shaving depth can be regulated by the applied pressure and the cutting angle of the dermatome, according to feel and the conditions encountered at the bottom of the wound. Tissue is shaved off until better-perfused tissue becomes visible and significantly less indurated tissue can be palpated.

Since the surrounding sclerosis is also removed (" fibrosectomy"), the shaved area is always significantly larger than the ulcer (Fig. 34.1c); in circumferential ulcers (Fig. 34.3), the whole circumference of the lower leg is ablated. The depth of shave depends on the extent of the induration and goes no deeper than the lower leg fascia – which in the often massively indurated and caked-up tissue (dermatolipofascioclerosis) is not always easy to distinguish from its surroundings. CT or MRI can help to define the shave depth (Fig. 34.2).

Extensive bleeding from large areas is rare. It can be stopped intraoperatively by raising the leg and applying short-term compression with damp compresses; large epifascial veins that have been severed are ligated and a purse-string ligature is placed around perforator veins. Surgery under bloodless conditions is possible, but makes it more difficult to assess the bottom of the wound (even pattern of punctiform bleeding) during shave therapy. TLA, on the other hand, does not interfere with this assessment.

The defects produced are covered with split-thickness grafts (meshed 1:3) in the same session (Fig. 34.1d); the tighter the mesh, the faster the healing and the less painful the first dressing changes. The split-thickness graft is taken from the ventral, lateral, and/or medial aspect of the thigh of the diseased leg with an electrodermatome set at 0.4–0.7 mm. It is fixed at the wound margin with acrylate glue.

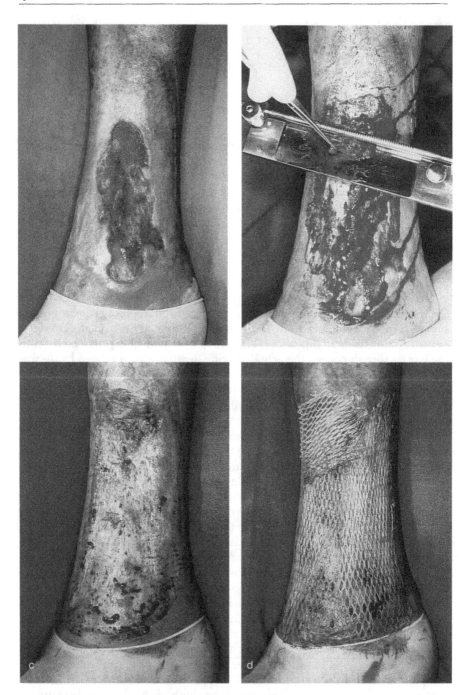

Fig. 34.1a–d. Technique of shave therapy. **a** Initial appearance; **b** extensive horizontal ablation of the ulcer and the dermatoliposclerosis using a manual dermatome; **c** appearance after shave therapy; **d** split-thickness graft at the end of surgery

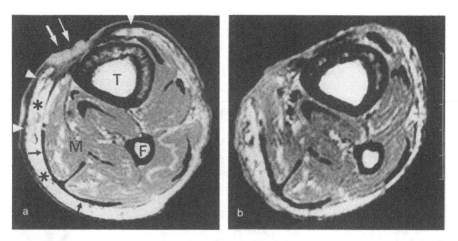

Fig. 34.2a,b. T1-weighted magnetic resonance images of the lower leg. **a** medial ulcer (*large arrows*), dermatoliposclerosis (*arrowheads*), subcutaneous tissue (*asterisks*), fascia (*small arrows*), tibia (*T*), fibula (*F*), muscle (*M*); **b** 2 weeks after horizontal ablation of the ulcer and the surrounding sclerosis and covering with split-thickness graft

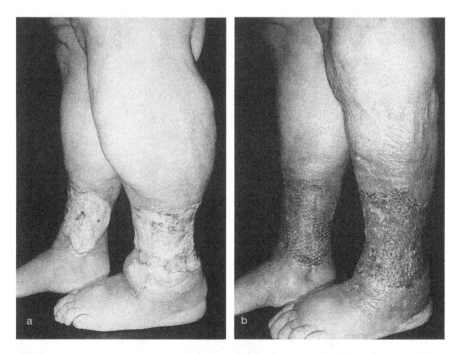

Fig. 34.3a,b. A 57-year-old woman with circumferential ulcers on both legs of 20 years' duration associated with post-thrombotic syndrome. **a** Preoperative appearance; **b** appearance 2 weeks after surgery

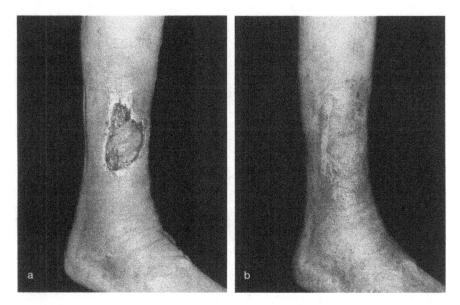

Fig. 34.4a,b. An 85-year-old woman with and ulcer on the right lower leg of 2 years' duration associated with primary main vein insufficiency. Marked calcification of the femoral and popliteal arteries without signs of vascular occlusion. **a** Preoperative appearance; **b** appearance 5 months after surgery

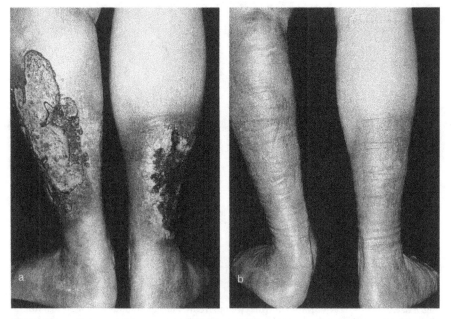

Fig. 34.5a,b. A 58-year-old man with ulcers on both legs of 25 years' duration associated with post-thrombotic syndrome. **a** Preoperativel appearance; **b** appearance1.5 years after surgery

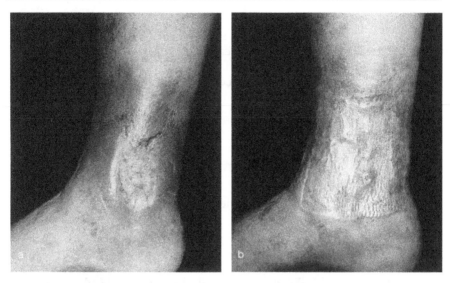

Fig. 34.6a,b. A 59-year-old man with post-thrombotic syndrome and arterial vascular occlusion of the lower leg type. Angiography showed occlusion of several centimeters of the proximal portion of the posterior tibial artery together with a long stretch of occlusion in the whole distal lower leg area; 8-cm occlusion of the anterior tibial artery in the distal part of the lower leg; 1-cm high-grade stenosis of the fibular artery in the middle of the lower leg with distal hypoplasia. Pressure values: dorsal artery of the foot: 130 mmHg; posterior tibial artery: 120 mmHg; brachial artery: 120/90 mmHg. **a** Initial appearance; **b** appearance 3 months postoperatively

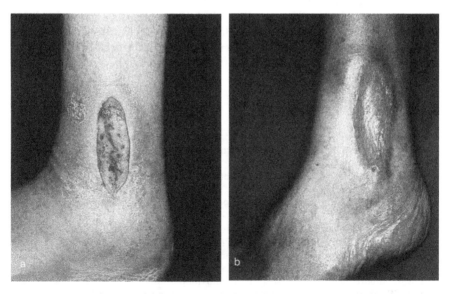

Fig. 34.7a,b. A 76 year old man with an ulcer of 5 years' duration associated with arterial occlusive disease of the thigh type. Pressure values: dorsal artery of the foot : 110 mmHg, monophasic; posterior tibial artery: 100 mmHg, monophasic; brachial artery: 180/90 mmHg. **a** Initial appearance; **b** appearance 8 months postoperatively

34.3   Specific Advantages

- May be used in elderly patients with cardiac or pulmonary problems in whom general anesthesia is contraindicated.
- Relatively simple for the surgeon to carry out him-/herself.
- Assessment of the bottom of the wound is easier because there is less bleeding in the surgical site.

34.4   Specific Disadvantages

- Infusion of the TLA can be painful.
- Waiting period required until anesthesia takes effect.

Concluding Remarks

Shave therapy is a relatively simple, quick, and particularly effective surgical technique for persistent ulcer in patients with superficial venous insufficiency. Unlike paratibial fasciotomy, which is only effective in medial ulcers, it can be applied to ulceration in all locations. Concomitant peripheral arterial occlusive disease is no contraindication in our experience. Peri- or postoperative antibiotic treatment is unnecessary. Since conspicuous level differences on the leg do not arise with shave therapy, there is less of an obvious step from the surgical site to the surrounding area than is the case with ulcer excision and fasciotomy.

Thus, a method is available to all surgical dermatologists and phlebologists which has shown impressive short- and long-term results in otherwise refractory cases. It would be desirable for shave therapy, which can be performed under tumescent anesthesia in many patients with venous ulcers, to become widely used.

References

1. Brinckmann J, Acil Y, Tronnier M et al (1997) Altered X-ray diffraction pattern is accompanied by a change in the mode of cross-link formation in lipodermatosclerosis. J Invest Dermatol 107:589–592
2. Gaber Y, Schmeller W (1997) Adjuvante operative Therapie bei rezidivierender idiopathischer Livedo-Vaskulitis. Phlebol 26:95–99
3. Gallenkemper G, Bulling BJ, Kahle B et al (1996) Leitlinien zur Diagnostik und Therapie des Ulcus cruris venosum. Phlebol 25:254–258
4. Galli KH, Wolf H, Paul E (1992) Therapie des Ulcus cruris venosum unter Berücksichtigung neuerer pathogenetischer Gesichtspunkte. Phlebol 21:183–187
5. Hach W, Vanderpuye R (1985) Operationstechnik der paratibialen Fasziotomie zur Behandlung des chronisch-venösen Stauungssyndroms bei schwerer primärer Varikose und beim postthrombotischen Syndrom. Med Welt 36:1616–1618
6. Hach W (1994) Operative Therapie. In: Rabe E (eds) Grundlagen der Phlebologie. Kagerer Kommunikation, Bonn, pp 193–219
7. Kaufmann R, Vranes M, Landes E (1986) Dermatochirurgische Behandlungsmoeglichkeiten des Ulcus cruris. Z Hautkr 61:923–939

8. Kirsner RS, Pardes JB, Eaglstein WH, Falanga V (1993) The clinical spectrum of lipodermatosclerosis. J Am Acad Dermatol 28:623–627

9. Lehnert W, Winter H, Bellmann KP (1993) Radikale Ulkus-Narben-Faszienexzision bei schweren und schwersten Formen der chronischen Bein-Beckenveneninsuffizienz. Tagungsbericht der Deutschen Dermatologischen Gesellschaft. Zentralbl Haut Geschl Kr 162 (Suppl): 204

10. Leu HJ (1991) Morphology of chronic venous insufficiency – light and electron microscopic examinations. VASA 20:330–342

11. Mayer W, Jochmann W, Partsch H (1994) Ulcus cruris: Abheilung unter konservativer Therapie. Eine prospektive Studie. Wien Med Wochenschr 144:250–252

12. Pflug JJ (1995) Operative Behandlung des supramalleolären medialen Konstriktionssyndromes bei nicht oder schlecht heilenden Ulcera cruris venosa. Phlebol 24:36–43

13. Roszinski S, Koeser T, Wihelm KP, Schmeller W (1993) Untersuchungen der Oxygenierung von Dermis und Subcutis bei Dermatoliposklerose. VASA 22(4):297–305

14. Roszinski S, Schmeller W (1995) Invasive (intrakutane) und nichtinvasive (transkutane) Messung des Sauerstoffpartialdruckes bei Patienten mit chronischer Veneninsuffizienz. Phlebol 24:1–8

15. Schmeller W, Rosenthal N, Gmelin E, Tichy P, Busch D (1989) Computertomographische Untersuchungen der Unterschenkel bei Patienten mit chronischer Veneninsuffizienz und arthrogenem Stauungssyndrom. Hautarzt 40:281–289

16. Schmeller W, Gmelin E, Rosenthal N (1989) Veränderungen des Retromalleolarraumes bei chronisch venösem und arthrogenem Stauungssyndrom. Phlebol Proktol 18:175–181

17. Schmeller W, Maack A (1990) Multilokulaere Sauerstoffpartialdruckmessung ("oxygen mapping") an der unteren Extremität Venengesunder und Venenkranker. Akt Dermatol 16:181–186

18. Schmeller W, Roszinski S (1996) "Shave"-Therapie zur operativen Behandlung persistierender venöser Ulzera mit grossflächiger Dermatoliposklerose. Hautarzt 47:676–681

19. Schmeller W, Gaber Y, Gehl GB (1998) Shave therapy is a simple, effective treatment for persistent venous leg ulcers. J Am Acad Dermatol 39:232–238

20. Schwahn-Schreiber CH, Kirschner P, Hach W (1997) Die stadiengerechte operative Therapie des chronischen venösen Stauungssyndroms. Vasomed 9:134–142

21. Sebastian G (1994) Die Rolle der Hauttransplantation im Behandlungsplan venoeser (postthrombotischer) Ulcera cruris. Wien Med Wochenschr 144:269–272

22. Tronnier M, Schmeller W, Wolff HH (1994) Morphological changes in lipodermatosclerosis and venous ulcers: light microscopy, immunohistochemmistry and electron microscopy. Phlebology 9:48–54

23. Vanscheidt W, Peschen M, Kreitlinger J, Schoepf E (1994) Paratibial fasciotomy. A new approach for treatment of therapy-resistant venous leg ulcers. Phlebol 23:45–48

24. Welzel J, Schmeller W, Plettenberg A (1994) Dermatoliposklerose in der 20 MHz-Sonographie. Hautarzt 45:630–634

35 Local Anesthesia in Children

H. Breuninger

Until today, the use of local anesthesia in children was limited, first, by the painfulness of the injection, which is not tolerated by children, and, second, by the fact that their low body weight means that the maximum dose of anesthetic is reached with a very small volume.

With the very dilute solutions employed in TLA, the maximum dose ceases to be a problem, while the pain can be eliminated by the technique of subcutaneous infusion anesthesia (SIA). The slow rate of infusion in SIA is not painful, and the fact that the doctor can stay at a distance – because infusion is controlled automatically – has a very calming effect on the children. As a rule, small children are held on their mother's or father's lap (Fig. 35.1–3); older children can be read a story during the infusion. Our recovery room, which we use for long SIAs, is equipped with a video player, so that the children can relax watching a suitable video. In most cases, the use of Emla cream can be omitted if 30-gauge cannulas are used for the first surface anesthesia. There is no reason for not using Emla cream, though, to avoid even the slight pain of the skin puncture.

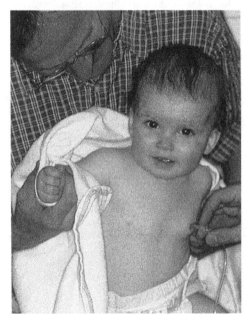

Fig. 35.1. A 6-month-old infant with a congenital pigmented nevus on the left breast to be ablated with laser. The necessary local anesthesia, administered as SIA, is tolerated without any problems

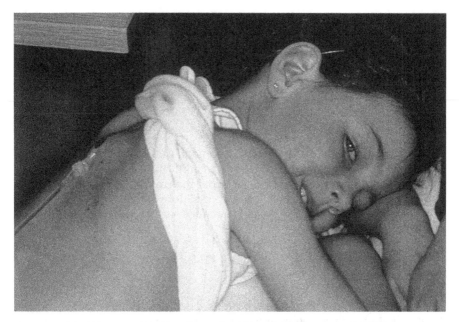

Fig. 35.2. This girl leans comfortably on her mother's knees during the automatic infusion

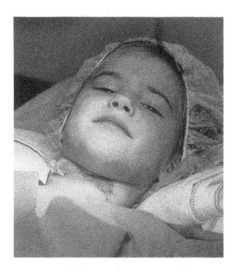

Fig. 35.3. This little boy is being read a story during the infusion

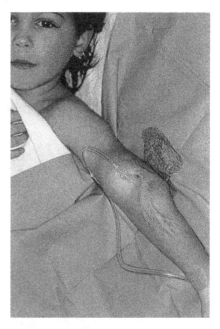

Fig. 35.4. After the painless second distal insertion of the 27-gauge cannula, this boy now looks fearlessly and trustfully at the doctor standing some distance away

This painless method of anesthesia usually wins the children over to such an extent, e.g., when they cannot feel the following injections in the partially infused area (Fig. 35.4), that they will also allow the subsequent surgery to be performed with complete confidence. Generous SIA followed by a sufficiently long waiting period (at least 30 min) is extremely important.

Premedication

In some cases, oral sedation with a diazepam analogue, e.g. flunitrazepam (Rohypnol) dosed per kilogram of body weight can be helpful (Fig. 35.5). For dermatological procedures Rohypnol is better than midazolam (Dormicum) because its effect lasts longer. In children, an oral dose of 0.03 mg/kg body weight is recommended (the solution, which is intended for intravenous or intramuscular injection, is given orally).

Prilocaine Dose

The maximum dose of the volume to be infused depends of course on body weight. In combination with epinephrine, which is indispensable in SIA, doses of 7 mg/kg may be considered to be totally harmless for a child at least 6 months old. This

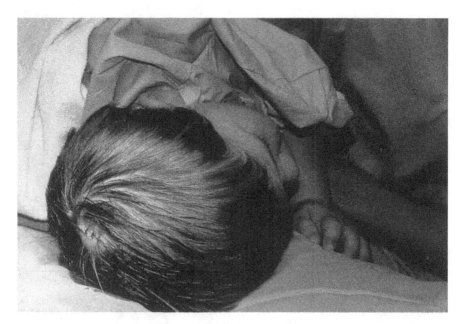

Fig. 35.5. In some children and for infusions in psychologically unpleasant locations, diazepam analogues (Dormicum, Rohypnol) can be very useful

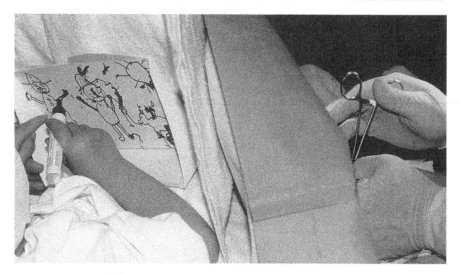

Fig. 35.6. Keeping children occupied and guiding them psychologically through the surgery is very important

means that, with a 0.1% solution, 6 ml/kg body weight may be infused – in a child weighing 5 kg, that is already 30 ml. Thus, the limiting factor is usually not the volume of local anesthetic, but sometimes the stress of a major procedure itself. In children below the age of 6 months, SIA can still be used, though with a reduced maximum dose because of the immaturity of the child's respiratory center. A particular consideration is the potential risk of methemoglobin formation. For very small procedures and in older children, the 0.2% solution with its faster onset of effect may be used.

Thus, SIA in children can often help to avoid the much larger undertaking of narcosis. Fasting and the prolonged postoperative observation needed after general anesthesia are unnecessary, which makes life much easier for the parents. In addition, the analgesia lasts much longer than in general anesthesia. Only after procedures near the maximum dose is postoperative observation required for 2–3 h because of the possibility of methemoglobin formation, but still without fasting. Our experiences with over 80 children have been very positive. We also treated 34 children with serial excisions of large congenital nevi. Only one of these children (6 months old at the time of the first procedure) manifested negative conditioning in the form of fear and aversion before the third procedure, so the following procedures were performed under general anesthesia. All the other children went along with what we were doing without any trouble (Fig. 35.6); some even said that they would be happy to come back for the next procedure.

Successful use of SIA in children, as in adults, requires some experience, and also sensitivity and and ability to empathize with the child and his or her basic fear of the unknown, which a child cannot control as well as an adult can. Not all children are suited to this procedure.

References

1. Arthur DS, McNicol LR (1986) Local anesthetic techniques in paediatric surgery. Br J Anaesth 58: 760–778
2. Arzneitelegramm 6/90, pp 52–53
3. Jöhr M (1993) Kinderanästhesie. Fischer, Stuttgart New York
4. Lund PC, Cwick IC (1966) Korrelation zwischen unterschiedlicher Penetration und allgemeiner Toxizität von Xylocain, Scandicain und Dylonest beim Menschen. Acta Anaesth Scand Suppl. 23: 475–479

Part A: Toxicity of Lidocaine in Correlation to the Plasma Level

Plasma level	Toxic symptoms
3–6 µg/ml	Subjective toxicity: paresthesias periorally and on the hands, restlessness, euphoria
5–9 µg/ml	Objective toxicity: nausea and vomiting, tremor, disorientation, muscular fasciculations
8–12 µg/ml	Seizures, circulatory decompensation
Over 12 µg/ml	Coma, respiratory and circulatory arrest

Part B: Possible Toxic side Effects of TLA and their Therapy

Side effects	Clinical symptoms and warning signs	Prophylaxis	Therapy
Methemo globinemia of over 20%	Cyanotic discoloration	Methylene blue (Tetramethylthionin) 1–3 ml/kg BW (or about 10 ml methylene blue 2%) i.v.	No prilocaine in risk groups: southern Europeans with glucose-6-phos-phate-dehydro-genase deficiency in history
	Headache	Vitamin C 2 mg/kg BW postop.	
	Restlessness	Thionine 0.2% (Catalysin) 10 ml i.v.	
	Dyspnea	O_2-application via a mask	
CNS arousal	Dizziness	O_2 application via a mask	Slow infiltration of the LA
	Fasciculations	2.5–10 mg diazepam (Valium) i.v	Speak to the patient during the infiltration
	Tinnitus		
	Fear		
	Nausea		
	Vomiting		
	Disorientation		
	Seizures		
Cardiovascular reactions	Bradycardia	Shock positioning	Pulseoximeter
	Decrease in blood pressure (depending on amount of TLA already used)	R-R-contol	
	Feeling of weakness	5 mg diazepam (Valium) v. or 2.5 mg midazolam (Dormicum) i.v.	Maybe ECG
	Possibly volume control		
	Sweating		
	Possible arrhythmias		
	Block signs		

Part C: List of Suppliers

3M Medical, St. Paul, Minnesota, USA, and, 3M Laboratories,
Gelsenkirchenerstr. 11, 46325 Borken, Germany
- Dressing materials, e.g. Coban

Astra GmbH, 22876 Wedel, Germany
- Local anesthetics, Emla cream

Byron Medical, 3280 East Hemisphere Loop, Suite 100, Tuscon, Arizona 35704
- Percutaneous sticks, ultrasound equipment associated with liposuction

Physician's Choice, Arizona, USA
- Personal hygiene, e.g. facial wash

Medi Bayreuth, Waldsteinring 6, 95448 Bayreuth, Germany,
medi@medi-bayreuth.de
- Compression stockings in standard sizes and also fitted, e.g., Struva 35

Wells Johnson Company, 8000 South Kolb Road, Tuscon, Arizona 85731–8230,
Internet: www.wellsgrp.com
- TLA infiltration systems and instruments for liposuction

E. Nehmad Intl.Petah Tikva, Israel
- 2 ml percutaneous stick, Multi-purpose 2-cc. MK 10

Novamedical Vertriebsgesell-schaft mbH, Am Seestern 8
40547 Duesseldorf, Germany
- Wound bandaids, e.g., suture strip

LaserPoint Nord-Süd GmbH, Hiberniastr. 6, 45731 Waltrop, Germany,
www.Laserpoint.de
- TLA infiltration systems and instruments for Liposuction

HK Surgical, 30280 Rancho Viejo Road, San Juan Capistrano, California 92675
- TLA infiltration systems and instruments for Liposuction